2-6-73

The Neuroses

A Psychoanalytic Survey

P. C. KUIPER M.D.

The Neuroses

A Psychoanalytic Survey

INTERNATIONAL UNIVERSITIES PRESS, INC.

NEW YORK

Library of Congress Catalog Card Number: 74–180732
ISBN: 0–8236–3555–4

Manufactured in the United States of America

CONTENTS

CONTENTS

1

GENERAL FOUNDATIONS

WE ARE in need of a psychology capable of providing insight into the psychic processes of the neurotic as well as into those of the healthy person. In search of such a psychology we examine man as an active member of the community of which he is a constitutent part.

As a rule textbooks like the present one begin with a long theoretical introduction. I do not condemn this procedure, yet I am inclined to accept Hegel's point of view, that the usefulness of a method is best demonstrated in its application after we have reached some depth in our investigation. There will be sufficient opportunity for some methodological observations. It seems expedient to proceed *in medias res*, and defer critical judgment.

Man's behavior, the sum of his actions, always takes place in relation to a given situation. German psychiatry of the last decades emphasized correctly that human beings should not be viewed in isolation from their environment, but observed in relation to it, just as a biologist observes the organism in relation to its environment. Man's environment is his community, the society of which he is a part.

The concept of adaptation which has proven itself so fruitful in biology is equally useful in our endeavor; however, the concept as we use it has a social context as well as a biologi-

1

cal one. Adaptation is an active process. We no longer use the concept as signifying passive submission to circumstances. On the contrary, adaptation implies that man alters these circumstances to suit his needs and wishes. We live in a world which in many ways is a result of man's own action, not nature in its passive state. The concept of adaptation shall be the point of departure for our further deliberation.

The question of what are the characteristics of a well-adapted action in its relation to the acting person may be raised. Our point of view is certainly phenomenological, but because of the many meanings attached to this expression we shall do well to use it with greatest caution.

To arrive at an action, we have to wish something to feel an impulse without which we cannot act. We act to satisfy our wishes and our needs. When we experience hunger, we eat, if a friend is ill, we send flowers or pay a call. Whatever we do, there is a motive for our actions. The word motive has a common root with the verb to move—there has to be something that moves us or else we do nothing.

A second criterion of adapted behavior is that it must be consonant with the demands of the society. A driver angered by damage to his car caused by another man's disregard of the traffic rules, and, in addition, angered by the behavior of the other man, may feel an impulse to attack the offender violently. The motive for such an action is understandable; yet, if the driver were to give in to the impulse it would be an inadequately adapted action. If instead he turns to the law, and the law proceeds to punish the offender and orders compensation for the incurred damages, his need to punish is satisfied without bringing him into conflict with society. This example demonstrates the second characteristic feature of adapted behavior: i.e., acting in consonance with societal norms.

We turn now to a third attribute of adaptation. Adapted behavior is in agreement with the norms of one's conscience. What society demands from us does not always coincide with the demands of our conscience. We may indulge in gossip and spreading of malicious rumors without being called to account by the police. We can arouse expectations in an attractive woman and later bitterly disappoint her without societal conflict. But most of us would not enjoy such conduct owing to the objections of our conscience. Conversely, there are activities prohibited by society, but condoned by our conscience. In spite of a no parking sign, we rarely hesitate to park our car there at night if the street is empty. We rationalize our behavior by claiming that the rule is flexible and applies only to the crowded daytime hours.

Thus, adaptive behavior is motivated by forces expressive of our individual personality. It is in conformity with the demands of society and also of our conscience. These considerations lead us towards formulations regarding the structure of the personality. The concept of personality structure will prove very helpful in further deliberation. We have termed the psychic agency, which judges our behavior and approves or disapproves it, the conscience. In psychoanalytic usage we refer to it as the superego and deem it a definite and dependable part of our personality.

We have as yet said nothing about the source of the strivings, needs and impulse. Freud named this source the id and we shall use this terminology. In talking about agencies of the mind we risk certain dangers. We are tempted to speak of superego and id as if they were concrete phenomena and we may give the impression of examining a rigid apparatus composed of separate clearly defined elements. Yet, fluidity and easy mobility is particularly characteristic for experiences in the inner world of the psyche.

William James (1899) referred to the stream of consciousness of thoughts and feelings. This notion was accepted readily and rightly approved in German literature. We must not think of superego and id as static things or substances, though they have a certain constancy, an enduring, permanent quality. The same strivings reoccur steadily and we listen to the same prohibitions and commands. These are as enduring as our wishes and impulses. Because some tension and conflict between our needs and our conscience is always in evidence, it is correct to speak of psychic agencies. Conflict presupposes opposing forces, forces which we ascribe to the agencies of the mind, which together form the psychic structure. We expect that our wishes, strivings and impulses, the voice of our conscience and also the demands of society, should give rise to a stable harmonious entity within us.

When such is not the case, efforts to bring conflicting factors into harmony are made. The attempt to resolve conflict is at times conscious, but it also takes place within us without our knowledge. We call this activity within the mind an integrating or synthetic function. To bring into harmony standards of conscience, demands of society and our impulses represents a difficult task, particularly when societal attitudes oppose our wishes. We have to resolve the engendered conflict somehow. We have assumed that we are familiar with the demands of society. But that is not always the case. Mentally deficient persons are unable to perceive with clarity the demands of their environment. Prior knowledge of societal norms can get lost, as in syndromes accompanied by dementia. Knowledge, the operation of the cognitive function, is a requisite for successful adaptation. We must be capable of acting on the basis of our insight and decisions. We also must have command of our voluntary motor functions. The functions which we have just enumerated—integrating or synthesizing, perceiving, and governing motor activity—we ascribe to a third agency: the ego.

We define the ego in terms of its functions, for the ego does not exist in a detached state. When we speak of the ego, we mean its functions. We are not surprised to find that one ego function may be disturbed while others remain operative. To learn how the various functions are correlated, we have to examine man in relation to his environment. While endeavoring to bring harmony between the wishes of the id and the demands of the superego and society, the ego must gather experience related to its environment and actively engage that environment in the performance of the ego's functions. It must take into account all the factors previously mentioned more or less simultaneously. The work required for that particular effort by the ego is called its synthetic function or integrating function. The concept of synthesis is used in the context of conscious psychic endeavor. We use the term integration in connection with unconscious mental processes, and biological processes.

We have not yet mentioned one important function of the ego, namely, reality testing. It is implied in the function of perception. To perceive is to discriminate. We have to discriminate between reality and fantasy. We may believe that someone is angry at us, and discover that we are in error. The following illustrates the significance of reality testing: A man believes that a woman he is in love with loves him in return. This however is not the case. Because of his false assumption he finds himself in an embarrassing and painful situation. In this case reality testing has failed, and the man has mistaken his fantasy for reality. The fantasy came about as a result of his wishes and expectations, not his observations. Whenever we act on the basis of such false assumptions we act unrealistically.

The ego, superego and id together form the personality structure. This structure must never be conceived as detached from its functions. They belong together, their existence is mutually interdependent. This is very often forgotten, and the personality structure is treated as if it were a mechanical apparatus, an engine. Such speculations remove one from the reality of life, and often are followed by failure to return to it. We must attempt to avoid this pitfall, and constantly keep in mind that we are not discussing material things, or organs, but structure and agencies which we define on the basis of functions and psychic forces. These provide the motivation for our actions. As we proceed, we shall discover that this structural model can perform splendid services for us in understanding man's psyche.

THE FUNCTIONS OF THE EGO

We have defined the ego as the central integrating agency of the personality. We may appropriately turn to a review of the ego's functions. We begin with the ego's relation to the world surrounding it. The ego takes note of its surroundings with the help of the sensory organs and of thought. Thoughts are sometimes referred to as "internal deeds" and there exists indeed a close relationship between perception and behavior in the external world. Fantasies develop into plans and these give direction for our actions. The ego distinguishes between fantasy and reality; reality testing is one of its functions. The capacity to distinguish between the internal and external world and between creations of fantasy and reality (which come about as a result of our wishes and anxieties) may get lost, as in psychosis. At times even the impressions transmitted by our sense organs cannot be distinguished from creations of our inner psychic activity, in which case we speak of hallucinations. Their presence always indicates a profound impairment of reality testing. Reality testing is a gradually developing function. An infant is not able to discern what happens within him and what happens in his external world. The world looks threatening to an anxious child—giants and witches populate the dark forest. He learns only slowly what belongs to his own body, and what is outside of it. The conscious awareness of "my body," and later, of "my ego and my self" develops but slowly. Reality testing remains a function subject to pitfalls; it fails easily, in adults as well as in children. Many believe themselves accused by others, when in fact they feel condemned by their own judgment. A young girl may feel pursued by men, but the basis for her fears or wishes may be in her own erotic needs. The young child's psychic structure develops along with his ego functions. Psychoanalytic psychology pays much attention to this development, and the study of psychic manifestations in the context of this development utilizes the genetic viewpoint of psychoanalytic theory. We shall do well to keep in mind the developmental aspects in examining the functions of the ego.

Thought capable of perceiving reality develops slowly; in the beginning thought establishes all kinds of correlations which do not exist in reality. At this stage we speak of magical thinking. Parents and people who deal with children have noticed that children favor rituals, and tend to adhere to certain unchanging sequences of behavior: The child insists that the doll be placed in the exact center of the chair, or else something evil is sure to happen. Magical thinking has an additional feature. In the child's fantasy it possesses great power, the power of a deed. The child fails to distinguish between thought and deed. A child, angry at his sister, may think: I wish I had another sister, a nicer sister. If, coincidentally, the sister falls ill, this is experienced by the child as a direct result of his "bad" thoughts. It is easy to see that magical thinking fosters the proliferation of intense guilt feelings. The incomplete differentiation between thought and action is also to be found in our neurotic patients. The omnipotence of thought causes the child to have feelings of guilt, but it also provides gratification: If my thoughts come true then it follows that I am very powerful.

In the course of growing up and through his experiences the child increasingly develops a growing capacity to distinguish between thinking and acting, between inner world and outer world, between fantasy and reality. He learns by experience. The ability to test reality and the adaptation to the changing conditions of reality are very significant aspects of intelligence. Intelligence can be defined as the capacity to learn from experience. Learning is connected with language to a very high degree. Perhaps there are thought processes without words or word symbols, but language is of the highest significance for the thought which enables us to adapt to reality. The child learns to speak, to master the language in his relationship to his parents. This implies that our recognition of reality also takes place within the relationship to the parents. It is a fact that the first perceptions of the external world develop on the matrix of an affective relationship. That is true also of the development of comprehension of the spoken word and the acquisition of speech itself. The child learns to perceive the need-satisfying person, to combine the partial perceptions impinging on him into a whole and he begins to recognize his mother. He becomes anxious when he fails to see the familiar person but sees someone else in her place. This anxiety cannot appear in the child's psyche prior to the capacity to distinguish the perceptions of the mother from those of another person. The fact that the development of the perceptive function depends on the affective relationship to the person attending to the child's need is of essential significance for the training and education of children. We may expect that the disturbance of this affective relationship resulting from the absence of a satisfying and constantly present mother figure will distort the development of the function of perception. Experience shows that this is indeed the case. But not only is the very young child's life influenced by affective relationships—we all know how much better the child of school age progresses when educated by a beloved teacher, or a revered master, and how rapidly the performance lags when conflict develops between student and teacher, or when the student dislikes his teacher. Attention to these factors would improve the process of education and make it more pleasurable to children *and* their teachers. At the beginning of life the affective gratifications are limited in scope. The infant is fed, fondled, warmed and moved about. He is the recipient of all these gratifications. We speak of gratification with a passive aim. However, very soon the child begins to obtain pleasure from doing something actively. He experiences pleasure when he moves about, and begins to undertake the exploration of his environment; he crawls, walks and runs. Activity, an active attitude, provides pleasure to the child. The drive impulses determine the child's curiosity and venturesome spirit, while the ego functions enable the child to turn his impulses into actions.

This brings us to a second group of ego functions: mastery of the motor apparatus, of the voluntary muscles and the sphincters. Exploratory activity in the course of which the child uses his motor apparatus is intimately associated with his getting to know the world around him. Reality testing is no more separate from the mastery of the motor apparatus, than from the affective gratifications of the drive impulses. It is similar to the adult who travels and seeks adventures to increase his knowledge. His adventures will leave impressions proportionate in intensity to the pleasure he gained from them. Perception and motor system, satisfaction of needs and learning have a close relationship to each other. Modern educational methods take these facts into consideration. Children are taught by being permitted to do things, and the learning process is facilitated through the awakening of the child's interest in what he is doing. An interested student can face the disappointing experiences unavoidably connected with learning. Development of the motor and cognitive functions is impeded by mothers who unduly restrain their children's activity. The result of a development so damaged is sometimes seen in the later life of these confined children. As adults they show little enterprise, not even in fantasy. They remain passive and inert even in the world of their internal experience, and their imagination is limited. They entirely lack the interest and gratification that comes from learning.

Let us turn to the ego's relations with the drive.[1] To learn to deal with one's instinctual impulses is a very difficult process. In the beginning the child is quite powerless in his relationship to the instinctual impulse. In a child that is left alone and experiences hunger we observe a mixture of rage, feeling of helplessness and anxiety; we deduce all of this from his behavior. What are the methods available to the ego in its relations to the drives? To answer this question we turn to the examination of adult behavior where the ego functions are move easily studied. When necessary for our discussion we shall turn our attention back again to the child.

We have referred to the drive without accurately defining it. It is time to define what we mean by the drive and by describing its characteristics and we wish to give the word a psychological meaning. Experientially the drive is characterized by tension perceived as displeasure; gratification of drive impulses on the other hand leads to pleasurable discharge of tension. We note the tension is completely unpleasant and painful only when it is not coupled with expectation of a pleasurable discharge, when the longing cannot be experienced as one that will be satisfied shortly. To use hunger as an example: The sensation of hunger is unpleasant, but we can derive pleasure from thinking about and imagining the forthcoming satisfying meal. We note still another characteristic of drive experience; we experience both tension and discharge as something physical. And now we return to our question, how does the ego of the adult deal with instinctual impulses, i.e., with needs, the source of which is the drive? We can control the need and keep it in abeyance, or we can turn it into an action designed to obtain its gratification. Let me quote an example: In the course of a journey a happily

---

[1] In the present volume *Trieb* is translated as "drive." When the text requires the adjectival form, "instinctual" is used, as in "instinctual life" for *Triebleben*. Tr.

married man meets a woman who arouses stormy emotions in him. He experiences an intense sexual desire for this woman, but he can control his desire. He is fully aware of his wishes, they are conscious wishes. In contrast, there are people who have the greatest difficulty in controlling their desires, they act upon them immediately though the situation may offer little inducement for direct action. Neither consideration for others nor the damage they are likely to inflict upon their own selves can halt their behavior. In such a case we judge the ego function concerned in the relationship of ego to drive to be feeble and inadequate. Psychopathic personalities have weak ego functions in respect to the drive. The functions of the ego can be damaged by disturbances of development, or by physical deterioration of the brain. In such instances men undertake actions which they would not have undertaken in other circumstances. Weakening of the functions of the ego are often a part of processes leading to dementia.

In addition to the drive impulses, the superego reactions also require meaningful and adaptive responses from the ego. Some people live under their superego's constant and compulsive pressure. They argue: "We must be honest under all circumstances." Honest to the letter, they inflict unnecessary pain on others. They talk when silence is the wiser course. They are unable to act in keeping with true ethical norms; they are compelled to obey every command of their superego and are unable to let consideration for others influence their behavior. In compulsive submission to their tyrannical superego they sacrifice their fellow man. The ego of compulsive people fails in its function to distinguish between adapted and nonadapted prohibitions and commands of its conscience. Generally we emphasize control of the instinctual impulses, but the capacity to control the commands of its conscience is no less mandatory for the ego than its drive mastery.

The ego has still other techniques to deal with instinctual

impulses and commands and prohibitions of the superego. They are not as transparent and as obvious as mastery and action, the techniques discussed so far. Again let us begin with a common situation: A man at work is unjustly censured by his boss. All day he feels slightly depressed. The following night he dreams that he hits his boss. During the preceding day he sensed no conscious animosity, he just felt out of sorts. If he had been asked whether he was angry, he would have said that he was not angry, just a bit disappointed because his work had not been appreciated. The anger then manifests itself in a dream. The psychic activity which results in the "disappearance" we call defense and we speak of defense against the drive. When we master a drive impulse, we are fully cognizant of doing so; when we use defense against the drive, warding it off, we do so entirely without conscious knowledge. Not only the drive but also the feelings associated with the drive are subject to the defense. It is well to keep that important fact in mind. Anna Freud (1936) called attention to this point in her book *The Ego and the Mechanisms of Defense*.

I would like to mention another illustration germane to this point because at first glance the concept of defense against the drive appears more difficult to comprehend than those activities of the ego which we describe as action and mastery. A married man pays court to a woman and obviously wishes to have an affair with her. But the woman has strong objections to a liaison with a married man and refuses him. One evening she sees a film in which a man embraces a woman and reaches for her breast. She is startled by the sudden realization that she sees herself in the moving picture engaged in an erotic situation with the man who had made advances to her. In this manner the erotic impulse asserts itself. In our first example, in which the ego warded off an aggressive instinctual impulse, although there was no immediate response to the painful event (the criticism by his boss), the depressive mood was a symptom formation. In the second instance, nothing at all occurred apparently. The instinctual impulse disappears with seeming permanence. In discussing the defenses against the drive we implied the presence of conflict within the personality. The conflict is between the drives and the ego. But the ego can also experience conflict with the superego. In such a situation we argue with ourselves, we seek our own advice. General usage assumes the existence of different structures in the personality. When they are not in conflict with each other we speak of inner harmony. The idea of harmony always requires the presence of more than one force in the psychical apparatus. Insight into intrapsychic conflicts played a significant role in the development of the psychoanalytic concept of structure.

We can now turn to further questions. How does the ego manage to keep instinctual impulses outside of consciousness? What faculties does the ego possess to ward off instinctual impulses and the feelings attached to them? The special functions used by the ego in the service of its extensive activity are also called defense mechanisms. Some authors dislike the word mechanism in connection with intrapsychic processes, but it is frequently used in the literature. We now proceed to a systematic discussion of these defenses.

MECHANISMS OF DEFENSE

Repression

One of the defense mechanisms most widely used, is repression. A repressed instinctual impulse appears not to exist. Sometimes such an absence is very disturbing and damaging for a person's adaptation to his life situation. Frigid women, incapable of experiencing sexual excitation and orgasm, have feelings of discontent and frustration which trouble them and their partners. Many marriages fail because of sexual difficulties suffered by one of the partners, although the relationship may contain many positive aspects. People who are unable to experience anger, who endure passively everything that is directed at them offer another example of the damaging effects of repression. In certain situations this attitude may appear as an adequate adaptation, as in the case of submission to an aggressive boss, but on closer examination we discover that the person suffers damage from the process of repression and fails in his general functioning. Such a person is adapted in a superficial sense, but not in the true sense in which we use the concept of adaptation. We may term this a *passive* adaptation.

Reversal into the Opposite

Most defense efforts do not cease with repression. The latter is often supported by other defense mechanisms. One could speak of relief forces deployed at threatened defense positions. Though this image is meant merely for purposes of illustration, it leads us to speculative considerations of psychic energy, which, from time to time, may prove useful. However, we shall adhere closely to what we are able to perceive and deduce from behavior and experience. We can also say that repression is too feeble, the drive impulse too forceful. Therefore the ego adds other defense mechanisms to repression. To speak of intensity of drive impulses and of feelings is to use a phenomenological description, for example, "mild" hunger, "raging" thirst, "deep" hurt, "intensive" longing. An interplay of forces occurs between the ego functions of mastery and defense on the one hand, and that which is being warded off on the other. In the terminology of our discipline we say: We observe the dynamics of psychic events, we apply the dynamic point of view.

At a later point I shall describe in a more systematic manner how the psychoanalytic theory is built up. At this time I shall enumerate the different points of view of the theory. When we explore the interplay of psychic forces we work with the dynamic point of view. When we are concerned with the relative quantities of the forces involved in the dynamics, we utilize the economic point of view. When we review the different psychic agencies which comprise the personality we speak of the structural point of view, and the topical aspect refers to separation into conscious and unconscious. The most fundamental point of view is the adaptive. We examine the events in the psyche in connection with the adaptation of the personality to the environment. But let us turn to the defense mechanism of reversal into the opposite. A classic example is the exaggerated neurotic concern for one's well being. A mother thinks constantly about her little son who is at school. She is tortured by horrible fantasies from which she is unable to escape. She imagines that the boy was hit by a car and is being brought home in an ambulance, or that he fell into the river and drowned. She is forever fearful that he will catch a cold and die of pneumonia. To protect him from these dangers she dresses him in heavy clothing while the other boys wear summer clothes; he must make a long detour to avoid the river; he must keep away from his schoolmates to escape being hit by a car at a crossing they customarily use, and so on *ad infinitum*. Such a son has indeed no easy life; yet we cannot claim that his mother is not doing her very best for him. How can we explain a behavior so futile and ill-adapted? We assume that along with her love for her child this mother has different feelings which are not in aggreement with her affection, and it is these discordant feelings that she defends against with her grotesquely exaggerated solicitude. Feelings like these are frequently inaccurately described and incorrectly understood, e.g.: "In fact such a mother hates her child; she hopes that he drowns or dies of pneumonia. Her hostility is evident in her burdening him with heavy clothing and forbidding him to play with his friends." The emphasis on the words "in fact" is most misleading. A mother who has the obsessive thoughts described here and whose behavior is so overprotective loves her child, and she uses her affection to suppress hostile feelings. She wards them off, hostility turns into exaggerated concern, a form of love results which is cruel to the child and tormenting for the mother. The mother experiences nothing of her hostility to the child or of her anger at him. If we were to let her know something of our theories about her behavior, she would respond with a sincere denial and protest: "I do not hate my son, I love him so much that I can never stop thinking about him. I could not live without him." We may say, the love and its manifestations are reactively stressed and enhanced in order to defend them against hostile feelings. But one correctly asks, why should a mother have hostile emotions towards her child? Some students become outraged on hearing our explanation for the overprotective behavior of the mother, and claim that it is disgraceful to assume that mothers hate their children. Of course there are many reasons which could cause a mother to have a hostile attitude to her child. A mother may regret having a child by a man she does not really love and take it out on the child. She may have married the father of the boy because she was no longer hopeful of finding a more suitable husband at her age, and because she very much wanted to have a child; she may have wished to get away from the drudgery of disagreeable work; she may love another man and want a son more like him. One can easily imagine such situations. These feelings of regret and annoyance towards her child escape her internal perception by means of being turned into their opposite. As happened in our example such internal conflict can result in the formation of a symptom. This woman suffers from obsessive thoughts; in other cases character changes could also result from such internal conflict. Some people are excessively compliant or timid in order to ward off the rage which they would experience if their hidden feelings were exposed. Supported by the example just discussed, I shall enter upon a closer examination of the dynamics of neurotic symptom-formation. A neurotic symptom has a defensive aspect, in this case the mother's excessive protectiveness and worry, and also a drive aspect, a derivative of the drive being the hostility. According to the formulation most frequently used the symptom is an unsuccessful compromise between defense and drive. We can recognize both components in it. We find something of the drive also in the corresponding affect. The excessively protective mother torments her child by her attitude, but her conscious intentions are the very best. We cannot say the same of her unconscious intentions. It is imperative that we distinguish sharply between conscious and unconscious intentions.

Another expression used to designate the defense mechanism of reversal into its opposite is reaction formation. We could use this expression but it is not advisable since the first designation makes what we mean considerably clearer. The word compensation can also be used. But compensation is also used to designate a conscious mental activity. The use of the same word for two different phenomena tends to lead to difficulties. The attitudes of the preachers and moralists also illuminate the defense mechanism of reversal into its opposite. These people constantly exhort others about their bad sexual behavior, they are always outraged, yet they themselves are forever preoccupied with sex. The warded off drive asserts itself in the very same behavior which was intended to ward off the drive. All these defensive maneuvers are not expedient. In the service of healthy adaptation, we use mastery; defense belongs in the realm of pathology.

Projection

Repression can also be bolstered by the mechanism of projection. Two defense mechanisms are used when repression alone is insufficient since the intensity of the instinctual impulses does not diminish merely by their removal from consciousness. Projection is present when we discern or believe to discern something in others that we cannot perceive in ourselves. A good example of projection is morbid suspiciousness. The suspicious person believes that others constantly conspire against him, are angry at him, or are offended by him. The person who projects has hostile feelings towards his fellow men; he is enraged at them or feels ill-used, but he is totally unaware of these reactions. We can find examples for each defense mechanism in the inner experiences and the behavior of people who ward off both sexual and aggressive impulses. These strivings are the cause of difficulties for them and they endeavor to remove them from consciousness. Therefore not only aggressive impulses but also sexual wishes can be subject to projection. A girl believes that people look at her in a suggestive manner. She mistakes the call of a thrush in the park for mens' whistles directed at her. She experiences as forbidden her own sexual desires awakened by a chance encounter with a young man and believes she recognizes the same desires in him.

We have previously pointed out that defensive functions are directed not only against drive impulses but also against our conscience. We can repress the voice of our conscience, or project it onto others. We believe ourselves accused by others when in fact we accuse ourselves. In the case of projection it is particularly easy to demonstrate the detrimental effect of this defense mechanism on adaption. A person who is convinced that his companion has malicious thoughts will reveal his suspicions in his own behavior and thereby disturb the relationship. We need the knowledge of the mechanism of projection to understand such processes taking place in society as racial hatred, which allows us to maintain that it is *others* who are bad, mean, unrestrained, and oversexed.

Why do we ward off our feelings? What is the meaning of these efforts? Since defense mechanisms are poorly suited for healthy adaptation, it must be asked why the ego deals with the drive and the demands of conscience in so unsatisfactory a manner. The answer is of particular significance for our understanding of psychology. We use defense mechanisms because the entry of drives or their derivatives into our consciousness tends to mobilize intense anxiety. The defense mechanisms are put in motion in order to avoid anxiety. We can illustrate this with the cases already mentioned. The man reacted to his boss' censure not with anger but with vague discontent; his rage appeared later in his dream. The application of the genetic point of view enables us to see why the drive impulses and related affects evoke anxiety. The little boy cannot permit himself to feel enraged at his parents, or acknowledge the desire to hit them, much less act upon such wishes, since he is completely dependent upon them. He will do everything to retain their affection and to remain certain of their love. Many parents punish their children by measures which evoke anxiety. Even verbal punishment may cause intense anxiety and anguish in the child: When I was growing up some parents frightened a child who tried to hit back by telling him that his hand would grow out of his grave and everybody would see that he was a child who wanted to hit his parents.

The words "wanted to hit" are of crucial significance. Not only the deed itself, but the thought of the deed, the intention alone is equally damnable. The belief that not only deeds but also thoughts and feelings are prohibited is common among educators and among religious groups. Deeds and thoughts are equally sinful. The child learns to bury the "bad" thoughts. Defense mechanisms are stimulated by education with its demands on the child. If parents explained to their children, "You are angry now, that is natural, but you have to learn to master your anger," the number of neurotic and more seriously afflicted people in the world would possibly be smaller. We should teach our children how to manage their impulses and feelings instead of stimulating the development of defenses. It is useless to reproach the parents for their attitudes in child rearing, since it is their own anxiety, the fear of their own drives which forces them to treat their children the way they do. In applying a psychological point of view we do not seek to place guilt, but to uncover the factors which explain to us the behavior and the feelings of people. This knowledge then enables us to suggest and assume measures of prevention. There is no doubt that sensible training, more appropriate than commonly practiced might prevent the development of many neuroses. With reasonably sound and healthy rearing, a child's anxiety could be replaced by confidence. Parents should learn to recognize neurotic reactions in their children as early as possible.

In summary: Defense activity is mobilized by fear of one's strict conscience, of one's drives and the feelings associated with them. These factors are of greatest significance for our understanding of psychic dynamics: anxiety is the signal for the ego to mobilize defense activity, anxiety is a nodal point in symptom formation and in character deformations. We find this observation confirmed daily in our psychoanalytic work. In the course of psychotherapy, patients learn to manage their anxiety; they discover through experience that as adults they no longer have to fear what frightened them when they were children. When anxiety diminishes, so does the intensity of the defenses, and the neurotic symptoms and character deformations become accessible to amelioration.

Let us return once more to the defense mechanism of projection and why it is employed. The projection of our own impulses seems a gain: We need no longer fear our own rages; we are protected from disappointment and discontent which trouble us because of sexual fantasies of which we are ashamed. The responsibility always rests on someone else. If we examine the situation more closely the gain reveals itself as fictitious, while the loss proves to be very real. We distort our self-image, we think ourselves better than we are, we fail to learn to manage our lives because we do not learn to know our own selves. Our social relationships are disturbed because we think that others are more hostile than they are in reality. Obviously, projection is an inadequate solution for internal conflict.

Displacement

A further commonly used defense mechanism is displacement. Displacement occurs, for example, when we are very angry at someone, but do not fully acknowledge it in our own minds, but instead direct our anger at a different person. A common incident is used to illustrate this: A man has an argument with his wife at breakfast, he does not assert himself, he is inclined to let her have the last word, because he is fearful of losing her love, fearful of being rejected by her, of being refused sexual gratification, or even of losing her altogether. Later, having arrived at his office, the secretary brings him the mail and he suddenly has a furious outburst at her. The fury that in reality was meant for his wife appears in relation to another person. Such a man can express anger only at those who cannot reply to his aggression. He is incapable of defending himself against those who attack and injure him. We are accustomed to seeing this mechanism in men we refer to as henpecked husbands.

Displacement of suppressed anger occurs not only as displacement to others but also as displacement to our own person, and we then become a victim of our fury. An illuminating example of this behavior can be seen in children who cannot express their rage at the person who caused their pain. They would like to attack or hit their parents but instead they destroy a doll or a toy of which they are particularly fond. Adults, too, show similarly unreasonable reactions. Let us think of a man who has just acquired a new bicycle. It is an expensive machine, rather too expensive, as he later reflects. So he pedals along the canal at dusk, a police officer stops him and serves him with a summons because his new bicycle has no rear light. His pleading and arguing is of no avail. He becomes so furious that he throws the bicycle into the canal, exclaiming loudly: "There, that is that." It is easy to see that in reality he wanted to toss the policeman into the water. The defense mechanism of turning against oneself is unusually dangerous. If the waves of rage become too stormy and this defense is used, the person can indeed burst forth in a frenzied attack on himself and even commit suicide.

Before we learned to consider unconscious motives and the functions of defense, such behavior defied understanding. Now it becomes clear to us that suicide is an expression of rage, though the person contemplating suicide is much more conscious of grief and misery than of rage. We shall see later that suicide is motivated by a combination of factors, but in each case one of the factors is the rage directed against oneself. We can take our life, but we can also destroy our enjoyment of life, our happiness. We can do away with our body, but we can also put an end to our experience of everything that makes life worthwhile. When the defense mechanism of displacement is used in this way its consequence is depression. The sufferer from depression effectively spoils his life through the aggression directed against his own self. We emphasize again that this technique of the defense is not subject to the conscious will; it is entirely unconscious. We deduce from the resulting consequences what processes take place in a personality which has become the victim of a defense like this. The person uses the defense mechanism and is simultaneously its victim. The defense used by the ego in depression has also been described as introjection of hostility.

It appears more accurate to me to reserve the concept of introjection for those processes which occur in the course of the development of the personality, and to speak in the case of depression of turning of aggression against the self. So far we have limited our discussion to the displacement of rage and anger to another object. One can certainly raise the question whether the same obtains for libidinal impulses, whether it is possible to displace feelings of love to which one cannot give expression on oneself. I believe that this is by no means impossible. We meet people who are unable to love others, and who take themselves as an object of unceasing attention. We then refer to their narcissism. Narcissistic people love themselves excessively. We must not however, miss the defense aspect of such an attitude. These people are wrapped up in themselves in order to avoid the need to love others; to love is impossible for them because of the strict prohibitions of conscience which inhibits their libidinal strivings.

Repression of Affect

A defense mechanism readily observable in obsessive patients is the repression of affect while the ideational content to which the respective emotion is related remains in consciousness. True repression removes not alone the affect from consciousness but also the experiences, ideas and thoughts which gave rise to it. A hysterical patient aroused while flirting with her boy friend entirely failed to notice her friend's sexual excitation. An obsessive-compulsive patient would perceive the man's excitation, but the corresponding emotions in herself would be entirely missing. Therefore, the patients afflicted with an obsessional neurosis or an obsessive character structure are to a high degree given to rationalization. They talk about emotional issues as if these were intellectual problems. I shall return later to a discussion of these personality types; they are the theoreticians of living. Some analysts write in these cases of isolation of affect from content, others prefer the term repression of affect.

Included with the defense mechanisms are also the mechanisms of "disavowal" [2] and "undoing." We speak of disavowal when a person cannot perceive or understand something because he is reluctant to have some events and circumstances enter his consciousness. Were that to happen, unendurable anxiety would result. Occasionally disavowal resembles a protective mechanism in the service of adaptation. A patient denies the malignant nature of his illness. In other instances denial leads to disturbances in the adaptation, as for example in a person denying the perception of the malicious character of his sexual partner. As a rule disavowal and repression act in unison. Mostly we use the concept of disavowal to denote the removal of perceptional contents from consciousness. Undoing means to abolish an action by way of executing another action of an opposite nature. For example, someone wanted to hurt another person, and instead sends him flowers to make amends for the hostile wish. I prefer not to include this behavior among the mechanisms of defense, but to consider it as one of the techniques with which we deal with our conscience. Using the structural model of the personality we can also state that undoing is one of the techniques used by the ego in its relations with the superego. Since we do indeed have to get along with our superego, this description is phenomenologically justified.

Regression

We conclude the discussion of the defense mechanisms with a description of the complicated process of regression. Understanding of the phenomenon of regression and its

---

[2] Disavowal and denial are often used interchangeably in the psychoanalytic literature. Disavowal is the preferable term. Tr.

consequences is particularly important for our comprehension of psychic events. Many students of psychology and psychopathology who strive to think in genetic and dynamic terms, do so without much success, because they lack sufficient knowledge of the symptom-formation, the character changes and the neurotic maneuvers which occur as a consequence of regression. We shall do well to distinguish two processes:

1. *The regression of ego functions, resulting in the loss of already established ego functions.* One can observe this in the case of children who have experienced a frustration. For example, a child who is successfully toilet trained, begins to wet and soil when the parents go away temporarily and leave the child in care of strangers.

2. *The regression of drives.* The regressed person falls back upon forms of drive gratification which are no longer appropriate to his present stage of development. For example, a timid young man who has a sexual affair with a young woman is then rejected by her because he was not dashing enough. The young man's response to this frustration is excessive masturbation. He resumes a form of sexual gratification customary in adolescence. A regression of his instinctual life has taken place. Such a regression is often accompanied by a partial regression of ego functions. We can easily imagine that the frustrated young man's work declines, that he has a tendency to withdraw from the world and to sleep long hours. This, too, is a sign of instinctual regression. Drives with passive aims then predominate over drives with active aims and passive gratification is sought at expense of the satisfactions of activity. The manifestations listed here are also the result of ego regressions. We shall discuss later that the ego is always affected in neurotic reactions, although the degree of its involvement differs widely. The examples we so far mentioned do not as yet clearly demonstrate the defensive function of regression. This has to be deferred until we

discuss the psychopathology of the different neuroses. We shall then examine the matter in detail. Here we limit ourselves to drives with a passive and an active aim. Some men are excessively passive in their social and sexual relationships because active conquest would mobilize their aggressive fantasies. Passivity and passive behavior, like the infantile dependent attachment they resemble, are regressive manifestations, which serve to ward off aggressive impulses.

Some General Remarks about Defense

We pointed out at the beginning that we have to consider together the instinctual aspects of the personality, the superego and the ego functions. The examination of defense processes showed that they have the task of keeping certain impulses out of consciousness. The defense processes influence the person's relationship to the external world. They imply a changed attitude to it. The agency responsible for this attitude is, as we have seen, the ego. Projection, for example, is a defense mechanism which displaces instinctual impulses and the feelings attached to them from the person onto someone on the outside: "I am not angry at him; he is angry at me." The perception of the external world is thereby affected adversely. The ego distorts reality and misperceives the intentions of other people as more hostile than they really are. An opposite response occurs when people cannot recognize the contribution of others to their misfortunes, instead ascribing the responsibility for all possible miseries to themselves—accusing themselves and idealizing others. The reality testing is disturbed in both instances. We must now examine the consequences of all defense mechanisms for adaptation. The hysterical patient in whom repression predominates has no insight into the sexual life of the people around her; she distorts reality in a way peculiar to her. We always must keep in mind that the defense influences not only the realm of instinctual life but that it at the same time causes a reality distortion. It does that by disturbing the ego functions which take part in the defense processes. We shall return to these problems in connection with the psychopathology of specific neuroses.

Knowledge of the defense mechanisms is indispensable for the understanding of the neuroses. Anna Freud has the distinction of having given us a systematic description of the defense mechanisms. We must recognize clearly that every psychic function, every experience, every defense activity can be in the service of warding off instinctual strivings and anxiety-provoking threats from the superego. It is not always possible to ascertain what the defense is directed against. An example will illustrate that fact better than a long theoretical explanation: A married man of about forty has a series of sexual relationships. The first of these extramarital affairs had a particular significance for him. As he struggled with doubts and could not decide whether to stay with his wife and children, or leave them for his lady-friend, the lady married another man. There followed a series of amorous adventures which led to his divorce, but not to a satisfactory new marriage, not even to a gratifying love affair. Closer study clearly reveals that this man's most important inner problem is not sexual at all, instead it is a problem of his most intense competitive urges. His adventures had the task of warding off feelings of violent jealousy which were closely associated with fantasies of grandeur. His affairs could not provide satisfaction for him, since problems of rivalry and jealousy cannot be resolved through sexual adventures. Only the bringing of unconscious competitive needs into consciousness, and a reality-adapted gratification of the need to be something special can provide that resolution.

The reverse pattern is also possible. The defense against sexual problems then uses the means of aggressive activity. An example illustrates this behavior: A very ambitious man, driven by an enormous need to succeed, makes life very difficult for himself and for others because he cannot tolerate other people's knowledge and accomplishments. The frantic pursuit of success can never come to rest because of its defensive function. The pursuit of success wards off the deep dissatisfaction in his marriage to an older unattractive woman and the compelling concern with young and pretty women which preoccupies his inner life. Every libidinal expression can serve the purpose of removing different strivings from perception, and the same obtains for aggressive impulses. It is quite possible that a given kind of libidinal gratification serves to ward off the longing for another kind. For example, a particularly passionate man, whose sexual cravings are never satisfied, comes close to destroying his marriage by excessive sexual demands on his wife, of whom he expects permanent sexual submission. In reality, he seeks gratification of an entirely different longing: He wishes to be looked after, taken care of, provided with security; in short, he craves what Freud calls the gratification of drives with a passive aim. One could also speak here of a reversal into the opposite. The excessive sexual activity is a means to ward off the needs which we have just enumerated. We must recognize the fact that all manner of expressions, attitudes and neurotic maneuvers serve to conceal from our own awareness and that of others the perception of strong unconscious conflicts. These conflicts are very different from our manifest conscious problems. The knowledge of the operation of the defense mechanisms is furthermore indispensable for our understanding of dynamics, fully comprehensible only when we connect the dynamic and the genetic points of view. Anxiety is always the most fundamental motivation for the defense process.

The child's impulses which give rise to anxiety induce defense activity. Instinctual impulses are connected with infantile fears. Neurotic anxiety is characterized by irrationality. Instinctual strivings are no longer in reality dangerous to the adult; they appear dangerous only because infantile fears remain attached to them. The child had good reasons to be anxious—he was unable to cope with the drives and feared losing the love of his parents. The examination and treatment of a neurotic patient should at all times consider the analogy with the child. For this reason alone the training of the psychiatrist should include child psychiatry. It is important to keep in mind the fundamental significance of anxiety and its components, the fear of instinctual impulses and the fear of the superego with its roots in the earlier fear of the parents.

We must further note that the use of defense mechanisms becomes habitual in time, and the defense attitudes acquired in childhood and adolescence possess a certain constancy. Reich (1933) emphasized the significance of the defense processes for the formation of character.

I would like to recall to the reader's attention the overprotective mother in order to demonstrate once again the difference between symptom and character defense. The mother's obsessive preoccupation with her child is a symptom, an inappropriate compromise between defense and impulse. She suffers because of it, she experiences her symptom as ego-alien. A person's excessive solicitude can also represent a character trait and this is experienced as belonging to one's person. The character trait is ego-syntonic, and is permanent. We can say, it is a part of the structure of the personality. The neurotic defenses are relatively invariable, they are a structural component of the personality. In cases of psychotic deterioration we observe the failure of the defense. Anxiety follows, and instinctual impulses inundate the personality. Certain patients employ a defense pattern which has little structure and little constancy, they alternate between different forms of defense. We see this in neurotic patients with a weak ego, also described as borderline personalities. Occasionally these patients distort reality to an almost psychotic degree. Their reality testing has broken down.

Their anxiety is always more or less conscious, and their defenses are inadequate for their purpose.

SUPEREGO AND EGO IDEAL

Let us now turn to the superego. One often hears the question, why are children disobedient? I believe a more appropriate question is, How does it come about that children mind us at all? Children want to follow their impulses and not the rules that we prescribe for them; it is amazing that children learn to accept the commands and prohibitions of adults.

An inquiry into the reasons for the child's capacity to become obedient can be advanced by a genetically and dynamically oriented psychology. We learn that the child obeys his parents because he does not want to lose their love. There exists a powerful emotional bond between child and parents; in the case of the very young child, between him and the mother. The child foregoes the gratification of certain needs in order to secure the approval and love of his parents. We conjecture that this attitude is based on a biological necessity, since the child is totally dependent on his parents' support; he could not survive being abandoned by them. The human child is dependent on this support much longer than the young of any other living species. It is therefore natural to think of the biological root of the child's fear to lose his parents or his parents' love, i.e. self-preservation, which may be considered a primary life instinct. Some educational systems quite openly threaten the child with abandonment. No longer to be loved by the parents implies the threat to be sent away, to be abandoned, e.g., "If you don't behave we shall give you to the gypsies." Possibly such threats are a thing of the past. However, I should like to caution those interested in psychology against undue optimism in this regard. The child feels secure as long as he senses the parents' love and he feels threatened when he observes that the parents are angry and are critical of his behavior. Therefore the child complies with the parents' wishes even when complying requires a sacrifice on his part. In short, fear of the loss of love is the child's motive in obeying his parents, and that circumstance leads to the formation of the superego. At first the child pays heed to the commands and prohibitions only in the presence of the parents. Later their presence is no longer required for his obedience. It is as if the parents had become a part of his person, and even though they are physically absent their voice speaks to the child from within himself. What happened here we designate as internalization. Phenomenologically this is a fitting description. Everyone subject to a conflict of conscience knows from his introspective personal experience that he carries on a dialogue with himself. He converses and argues with himself. Consider the following internal conversation: "Should I go swimming today or visit my sick cousin instead? I should call on him . . . who knows how long he is going to live . . . it is most unkind of me to show as little concern for him as I have shown recently. We used to play together and have so much fun." Then another voice: "Yes, but must I always sacrifice my free time for such matters? I looked forward to this day of swimming, after weeks of hard work. Have I no right to enjoy myself and have some leisure? Am I demanding too much in claiming one free day for myself?" Sometimes the solution to the dilemma sounds somewhat like this: "I cannot abandon my wife and children on such a beautiful summer day, my duty towards my own family must come first. I see so little of the children." A solution is sought which will assuage the conscience. One neglects one's duty and yet emerges from the conflict as a kind father and benefactor of one's family. Fortunately man is quite often capable of listening to the voice of his conscience, and to serve the interests of others along with his own.

Clinical experience and self-observation show us that the personality contains several elements which converse with each other. As children, we carried on similar conversations with our parents and we continue them with ourselves in later life. If our relationship with our parents was friendly these conversations could have been very pleasant and helpful, and for the most part a solution was found which satisfied all parties. If, however, we had tyrannical parents, our superego also frequently acquires a tyrannical character. In such instances the development of a rebellious attitude towards the conscience may be observed. In people with a disturbed psychic development this attitutde can assume serious proportions.

The superego has two components: a prohibiting agency which frequently evokes anxiety, the superego proper, and a more benign component which is called the ego ideal. What are the specific differences between superego and ego ideal, and how do these agencies develop? We start with the assumption that the ability to form a superego is an innate quality. As we said earlier, the child takes into his own personality the prohibitions and commands of the parents, in order to preserve their love. He values that love more than the gratification of his instinctual impulses.

The ego ideal has a different source, it does not grow out of an internalization of the restrictions placed on drive gratification. Once again we shall give an example to illuminate the formation of the ego ideal: The little boy stands in front of the door. He wants to open it and enter the room. He tries to turn the handle, but his hands are not yet strong enough for that. The father arrives and opens the door without much effort. The little boy looks up with admiration to his powerful father. He, too, would like to become as mighty as his father whom he idealizes. The boy wants to be able to do everything the father does. One can observe this easily in children's play activity. The father can drive an automobile, the child directs his toy cars. What a mighty impression it must make on the little boy when he sees his father drive such a huge machine. He thinks, "I will be able to do that too when I become like father." *Mutatis mutandis* the same applies to the little girl. It may be her ideal to be able to cook for the father just as the mother does, to dress and make herself pretty like mother does, and also to care for little children. One can see all this clearly when she plays with her dolls. But the little boy cannot open the door, nor can the little girl cook and bake. The technical formulation for this psychic situation is as follows: The child forms an ego ideal because of narcissistic injuries. This is not as complicated as it seems. When he observes that he is unable to accomplish some task his self-esteem suffers. To undo the hurt, he resorts to the fantasy: some day I shall become a man like father. The little boy sees himself and evaluates himself not only as what he is, but also as what he wants to be in the future. The continuous juxtaposition of what he is and what he wants to be provides a healthy stimulus for his development.

We see that the ego ideal is formed not on the basis of commands, but on the basis of wishes: the fear of loss of love plays no part in its genesis. We conclude that the ego ideal is the healthier, potentially less dangerous of the two aspects of the superego. The ego ideal develops through the internalization of the kind and encouraging images of the parents. It is of great significance for a man's life whether the superego develops predominantly on the basis of commands and prohibitions or on the basis of the formation of ideals. The man guided in life by his ego ideal is fortunate; he sees his goal before him. But the man who is controlled by the superego is preoccupied by prohibitions. He constantly fears to transgress.

Let us imagine two young women: On the basis of her ego ideal, the first feels no desire for a sexual relationship with a man she knows only superficially. The second also has no

sexual wishes, but due to her excessively strict superego prohibitions. We expect that the first young woman is able to
accept a joyful sexual experience, but the probability is great
that the second woman is inhibited and unable to permit herself the experience of sexual gratification. The superego prohibitions are so intimately connected with infantile anxieties
that they prevent a wholesome adaptation. Experience
teaches us that children absorb the standards of their parents.
The children of puritanical parents feel guilty upon visiting
the cinema on a Sunday while other children enjoy the picture with an easy conscience. One cannot fail to take notice
of the relation between conscience and parents. However, we
frequently observe that children follow their own and not
their parents' norms. It is a fact that many persons are much
stricter in their attitude to themselves than their parents
once were. I should like to deal with the last point first.
What causes the superego to become so much more severe
and prohibitive than the real parents were? The attempt to
answer this question leads us to one of the most significant
subjects of the theory of the neuroses. The psychic processes
involved in the formation of conscience are by no means
simple. We cannot, therefore, give a single answer to this
question. Many factors contribute to the development of a
strict conscience. I should like to mention the most important factor first: A child confronted with a parental prohibition becomes angry. It is dangerous for the child to direct his
anger at the parents. The degree of the danger depends on
various circumstances. If the parents are very irritated the
child will suppress his anger out of fear that the parents' ex-
asperation will grow further which would increase the danger of losing their love. He gives up doing what he would
most like to do, i.e., express his anger by attacking the parents. How does the child manage the anger which he cannot
express? We mentioned in discussing the defense mechanisms
that the child turns the anger on himself. Continuously rag-

ing against oneself results in frustration and loss of pleasure in all activity. The theoretical formulation is that the super-ego becomes the carrier of the aggression provoked by the environmental prohibitions and commands. The superego acquires a hostile character; it is imbued with the hostility which was originally evoked by the parental prohibitions and was directed towards the parents. **1734610**

Certain educational measures compel the child to develop a severe superego. We must mention here particularly the attitudes which prohibit not only the open expression of hostility but even its experience in silence. The reactions of parents in this regard vary widely. A child is forbidden to play outside during rainy weather. The child is angry. In his anger he overturns some knicknack. One mother's reaction might be: "I can well imagine that you are angry because you can't play outdoors and you would like to break something, but please don't destroy something that is valuable." In contrast, another mother may react in her annoyance with loud reprimands: "Now why do you behave like this, is it my fault that it is raining today? You should not be angry, I thought you were a sweet, patient child, but you are a disappointment to me." When, as frequently happens, not only the expression of emotions is prohibited, but also the emotions themselves, the child is deprived of an opportunity to learn to manage them adequately. For example, when a little boy acquires a baby sister his jealousy is not mentioned, instead the family's injunction to him is to love the baby, be nice to it and not to aggravate mother by being jealous. The educational measures change with the times, but the attitudes described above are still quite common. A much better approach to the problem would be as follows: Certainly, you are jealous, but in future you will have much fun with your sister. There is still enough love left over for you, even though you must share it with her now. The prohibition of emotions leads to their repression, to defensive maneuvers; the anger generated as a consequence of frustration is turned upon the self, and there follows the formation of a severe conscience. The tendency of a child of lenient parents to turn anger against himself is not the only factor in the genesis of a stern superego. The child takes into himself the personality of the parents not as it is but as he experiences the parents to be. An anxious child experiences the environment as threatening, and these threatening figures then become a part of his own personality. Some children frequently experience their parents as angry; these angry parents then become internalized as part of the children's consciences. Think, if you will, of the monsters, the witches, and the giants, which dominate the dreams and fantasies of children. These anxiety-provoking figures frequently show features of the parents: The father makes huge steps like the giant in his seven-league boots; the mother prepares the food and gives candy, but the witch also dwells in a gingerbread house, and she can devour children. The malevolent figures can be introjected and become a part of the personality of the child. In later life these figures reappear in our nightmares. The image man forms of God also evokes anxiety. In psychotic conditions the patients are tormented by cruel, terrifying apparitions in which one recognizes the images of the parents. A child that has a good, trusting relationship with his parents will not be too disturbed in his development by the introjection of such anxiety-provoking figures. Our inner life is to a high degree influenced by the nature of our past and present relationship to our parents.

The experience of hostile parents is not the only factor to cause introjection of figures evocative of anxiety. Often the child thinks that his parents are much more wicked than they are in reality. He forms this idea on the basis of his own feelings. He thinks that the parents are irate and furious because he himself is furious. Children have strong instinctual urges, are easily frustrated, and react readily with rage. They perceive the parents as being as angry as they are themselves

—and eventually much angrier—because they use the distortion of reality as defense against their own rage. In the formation of a severe conscience, projection plays a significant role. The turning of aggression against the self leads to a strict conscience, or differently expressed, the superego becomes the carrier of the rage provoked by the environmental commands. The anxiety-provoking fantasy figures—the fairy tale witches and monsters—also contribute to the formation of the conscience.

Another process occurs which adversely affects the superego formation and is independent of the parents. A child who imposes many prohibitions on himself consequently suffers chronic frustration—he observes that others enjoy the pleasures which he foregoes. A group of children is playing in a puddle but the nice little girl abstains from joining them for fear of soiling her pretty and clean dress. Inwardly she is in a rage, which she experiences as being out of temper, as unhappiness, as a vague discontent for which she does not know the reason. Since she cannot rid herself of the anger, least of all express it against the parents, she turns it against herself and gets into increasing difficulties. Plato refers to Eros as a self-multiplying force. The same can be said of neurotic processes. They tend to increase steadily in scope and intensity. One wishes that parents were familiar with these processes and able to recognize them. Were that the case, the task of directing the development of children into wholesome channels would surely be easier than it is now. Unfortunately, we have not progressed that far—most physicians know nothing of these processes, and parents know even less.

The earliest stages of development contribute to the formation of the first primitive precursors of the superego. We shall return to them when we discuss the developmental stages in detail. For the time being the following considerations should be mentioned: During the first phase of the child's development instinctual strivings with a passive aim predominate, such as the wish to be cared for, to be fondled and fed; but soon the child's activity begins to develop, and much of his later well-being will depend on the attitudes assumed by the parents towards the unfolding infantile activity. If they prohibit too much and fail to provide opportunities for the child to discharge his energy, the child will absorb these prohibitions into his own person and develop into an inhibited, inactive youth. I have observed severe deformations of character in persons raised by mothers who have severely obstructed the activity of their children throughout early childhood. If these people ever undertook any activity at all, it was wholly without joy. They sought out the gratifications of instinctual tendencies with a passive aim, much to the detriment of their capacity to adapt to the requirements of daily life. They derived no pleasure from meaningful work, which for so many people is a source of intense gratification. Many parents are particularly strict during the stage of development in which children enjoy messing and smearing. They prohibit this activity and punish the child, although it is not difficult to guide the need to smear into tolerable patterns, for example by providing the child with sand and water, with clay, paint, and similar things. The harsh prohibitions which are taken up into the personality during this phase frequently congeal into a superego nucleus difficult to reach and often inaccessible to therapy.

The manner in which anxieties related to the genital phase influence the formation of the conscience will be discussed later. Most certainly the influence of this period is not always decisive. Frequently the decisive factors have occurred much earlier, and as a rule all different phases of development contribute their share to the disturbances of the superego.

Some people indeed fully internalize the commands; they acquire their own moral sense and henceforth follow their own ethical principles. Their moral judgment is independent of the opinions of others. Luther, who spoke the famous words, "Here I stand, I cannot do otherwise," is a good example of such a man. Complete internalization of ethical and moral precepts does not always take place. The capacity of self-judgment is in many people dependent on their judgment by others. When social standards change, so do the personal norms. What in reality is fear of punishment and ostracism is often mistaken for a feeling of guilt. An example: A young girl felt very guilty because of a sexual experience, but she quickly lost her guilt feelings as soon as her menses occurred at the proper time.

The psychology of guilt feelings is quite complicated. We begin with phenomenological distinctions. We often call something a guilt feeling which in reality is social anxiety, i.e., fear of an embarrassing situation. Injured self-esteem is also often mistaken for a feeling of guilt. People say, "How could I have done this," and mean, "How could I, as good a man as I am, have committed so bad an act." They have disappointed themselves, they are therefore angry and experience it as a feeling of guilt. A healthy feeling of guilt facilitates adaptation and provides a motive to rectify a perpetrated injustice.

The person who has a healthy sense of guilt regrets what he has done to others: A neurotic sense of guilt has its roots in the aggression against one's own self, in the infantile fear of punishment and in injury to self-esteem.

In connection with the psychoanalytic theory of the formation of conscience one hears the following remark: If the superego is a derivative of the parental attitude no one can render an independent judgment on what is good or bad, judgment being an automatic process. That is true for many, but not for all men. The genuinely adult person can manage not only his instinctual impulses but also his conscience. He can critically scrutinize the demands of his conscience, and acquire in time a different system of norms than that conveyed to him by his parents. The mentally mature person is no longer subject to the commands and prohibitions of his childhood. He will instead review the consequences of his actions, and will adjust his behavior accordingly.

From what we have said so far one could conclude that though a superego that has become too severe will have a disturbing influence on adaptation, the ego ideal under all circumstances develops favorably and always has a beneficial effect on the person's adaptation. That is not the case. The ego ideal too can play a disturbing role. We cannot state: The superego is always too severe; the ego ideal on the other hand is always a stimulating and encouraging agency. On the contrary, the ego ideal can also be disturbing and it can contribute its share to the genesis and the perpetuation of neurotic symptoms. When it is called upon to remedy all the injuries to the self-esteem the ego ideal can easily become too exalted and too rigid in its expectations. An ego ideal adapted to reality develops when the parents encourage and help the child; in such a setting the child can say to himself: "I shall be able to accomplish later what I cannot do now." The child speaks to himself as the parents speak to him, or, for reasons which we have discussed above, he is perhaps a little more strict with himself. But a child who is disappointed in his own performance and has to do without parental sympathy and comfort, will escape into fantasies. One can easily imagine such a child. He fails in some effort, and instead of being comforted and helped he may even be ridiculed. He begins to indulge in fantasies: "I can do everything, enter closed doors, lift up a house, everyone will have to listen to me." In his imagination the crowd of listeners will grow in inverse proportion to the number of those who at present pay attention to him. He will imagine he knows everything, mainly those things that are now being kept from him. Anger often lends a vengeful character to these fantasies of grandeur. This process extends far into adolescence. A girl forced to be a wallflower will day-dream that all men compete for her and seek her favor, but she refuses all of them. A young man, feeling that he is treated impolitely will see himself in his fantasies as the president of a huge corporation, treating his employees with disdain. The wrongs suffered stimulate the formation of an exaggerated ego ideal. We see here the same process that we observed in the case of the superego, namely that of an evil growing on itself: The higher the ideal, the less it can be reconciled with reality. Measured in terms of his fantasy the child is particularly helpless, and the adult who believes himself powerful in fantasy, feels keenly how limited are his accomplishments. The injuries to the self-esteem are compensated for in fantasy, the ego ideal grows more taut and inflexible, and reality is not at all in consonance with the omnipotent fantasies. We find these boundless and megalomanic fantasies again in the delusions of our psychotic patients. They have lost all touch with reality. Many neurotic and psychopathic patients do not attempt to fulfill their ego ideal in fantasy, but in vain try to do so in reality; in their case the ego ideal contributes not to delusional formations, but to discourgement and other disturbances of adaptation.

Let us review some further disturbances in the formation of superego and ego ideal. We have discussed the excessively severe superego and the demanding ego ideal. We saw that the processes of internalization depend upon the mutual relationship between parents and child. If that relationship was poor, disturbances are likely to occur. Hostility towards the parents has in its wake a defensive position towards their prohibitions and their moral and ethical demands, even though the parental origin of the superego and ego ideal is not consciously experienced. The person knows what he should do, or how he should behave, but he does not act upon his knowledge. He stands in opposition to the internalized images of his parents. We can observe this in neurotic and even more in psychopathic personalities. In some instances it seems as if a person has no conscience at all. In my opinion, conscience is never entirely lacking, but its voice is inaudible because of a profound deformation of the personality structure, such as occurs in children whose emotional needs were severely neglected in early childhood. The regulating function of the superego fails here entirely. The discontent of such people points to the disdain and condemnation they feel towards themselves. They suffer the pressure of their severe conscience, but they are powerless to adjust their actions to their demands.

A desperate situation results for the child when one parent praises what the other parent condemns. The father of an asocial family may encourage stealing while the mother may be most aggrieved by it. A child in such a family is at odds with himself when he steals, and has no inner peace when he abstains. Psychopathic patients describe the following conflict situation: "Decent behavior makes me feel like a weakling, but when I deceive people and take advantage of them I am a scoundrel." Neurotic patients have similar conflicts, for instance, in cases where one parent wants to bring up his child in accordance with norms rooted in orthodox religious beliefs, while the other favors a free-thinking view of the world, and encourages an experimental attitude to life. An old proverb saying that, "when two faiths sleep on one pillow the devil sleeps between them," contains some psychological justification. Unless the parents show much understanding for the child in his ambiguous position, and not only recognize what their differing attitudes mean for him, but also adjust their own behavior accordingly, he will have difficulty in gaining a harmonious attitude to himself and to others.

Analogous statements can be made about the ego ideal. It is very confusing for the child to grow up under the influence of contradictory ideals. The son who accompanies his father on hunting trips will have difficulty in forming a stable ego ideal if the mother has imparted to him an attitude of sympathy and compassion for all living creatures. The result in later years can vary. The boy can emphasize the pleasure in putting animals to death in order to silence his guilt feelings evoked by the maternal ego ideal. To ward off his aggressive feelings, he may turn into a rigid vegetarian, thus exaggerating the mother's ego ideal. Obviously the probability of a harmonious development is much smaller than in situations where mother and father are unanimous in their basic tenets and beliefs.

The ego ideal's lack of uniformity also has other sources than the internalization of differing parental images. These sources are inherent in the development of the ego ideal; they are a part of its dynamics. We see at times that one level of the ego ideal has features opposite to other levels. The well-behaved mama's boy discovers that in order to hold his own among his fellow students he has to to act boisterously and have amorous adventures. If he has a strong personality he will withstand the temptations; if, however, he harbors unconscious objections to his mother's teachings, he will adjust to his new environment without enjoying it. He remains unable to throw off the ego ideal inspired by his mother. Less fortunate than the snake, he cannot shed the skin which he has outgrown.

We see often that young people struggle with a weak ego ideal. People who have internalized contradictory sets of norms do not feel comfortable in life and are generally insecure.

One can also identify with parents whose own moral sense is unsuitable or inadequate. We call this a misidentification, an indentification with an unsuitable object. The following remarkable phenomenon is very frequently observable: Parents in modern families actually encourage their children to engage in improper behavior. A father, well-respected and an authority in his field, remarks to his son who has returned home with a bloody face: "I see you had a fight; that's fine, son, don't let anyone put anything over on you." This father had a puritanical upbringing, his mother warned him against getting into fist fights, but he wants to give his children a modern education. Often things are not as obvious, and one discovers the hidden connections only at closer examination of the circumstances. Johnson (1949) reports how she discovered that a child's truancy from school was obviously fostered by the child's father. The father had been a truck driver and now missed the occupation which had given him opportunity to move about the country. Prevented from roving himself, he now fostered his boy's inclinations to rove about. We ascribe significance not only to the parents' words and actions, but to the total parental attitude, particularly when it remains unconscious and finds expression in obscure ways.

How does the situation look when both superego and ego have developed normally? This is a difficult question because many investigators believe that the development of these agencies of the personality never comes to a conclusion. Yet, we can offer some statements about the adult conscience. A healthy conscience is autonomous and dependable; its contents are not determined by anxiety and defenses against unconscious libidinal and aggressive impulses. It is not determined by megalomanic fantasies designed to compensate for inadequate self-esteem. The ego makes the necessary decisions and does not forever listen to the interdictions of the superego. A person may say: "I know what I do and also why I do it." Here the viewpoint of adaptation proves particularly fruitful. He who has a healthy conscience asks himself: "Do I cause unnecessary pain to others by my action? Is what I intend to do good for the cause I wish to serve, or do the objective motives conceal more personal selfish ones?" A person with a healthy conscience is capable of being honest with himself.

We turn once more to the ego, particularly in reference to

self-esteem, the estimate of one's own value. We see that our self-esteem depends in large measure on our relationship to the internalized parental images. We do not feel that we are good when our conscience condemns us and when we do not meet the expectations of our ego ideal. The expression, not good, in this context covers several meanings: not happy, not satisfied, in ill humor, also not in good health, but the unconscious significance is literal: "I am not a good person, I feel condemned by my superego and not in harmony with my ego ideal."

Our mood is certainly influenced by our physical well-being, but undoubtedly also by our relationship to the psychic agencies which we have discussed in the foregoing. Psychoanalytic psychology has genetic and dynamic aspects. We applied both aspects in sketching the development of the functions of the ego and the superego. The study of the psychopathology of the specific neuroses will give us an opportunity to examine more closely some details.

THE DRIVES

We turn next to the development of the instinctual life. By addressing ourselves first to the ego, then to the superego and finally to the instinctual life, we introduce an artificial distinction. It is clear that the child develops as a whole, of which ego, superego and instinctual life are merely different aspects. If we keep that fact in mind we shall avoid erroneous conceptualizations.

Instinctual life, like the other aspects of the psyche, is subject to a gradual development. We distinguish the oral, anal, phallic and genital phases of development. Each phase has its own characteristic relationship to the respective objects of the drive.

What are the psychological features of the drive? The drive has a source in the areas of the body in which sensations of tension and relaxation occur which are also called erogenous zones. The drive has an aim, i.e., the satisfaction, such as satiation of hunger. Finally, the drive has an object as food does in the case of oral drives. The sexual drive has its erogenous zone in the genital organs, its aim is the experience of orgasm, its object the sexual partner.

The newborn infant begins his development with the oral phase, he experiences tension and relaxation of tension, hunger and satiation; he has the need to experience pleasurable sensations in the mucous membranes of the mouth, with and without the intake of food. We must not use the concept of orality too narrowly. The child in that phase also wants to be fondled, warmed, taken up and moved about. In the first months of his life the infant has no clear idea of the person gratifying his intensely experienced needs. This changes as soon as he begins to connect the impressions that impinge upon him with the vague images of the person attending his needs. He smiles at the mother and is anxious when faces of others enter his field of vision. After a satisfactory feeding an infant feels well and will include his environment into this feeling of well-being. During this phase of development a sharp distinction between him and his environment is still lacking. The feeling of satisfaction gives him a feeling of confidence in the world and in his own goodness. Even before the earliest object relationships have developed, the experience of basic trust provides the foundation for the child's subsequent relationships to his environment. It is, therefore, of great importance. When the infant is hungry or cold he submerges into a state of anxiety, rage and a limitless diffuse craving. This condition changes suddenly into a state of profound happiness, peace and satisfaction as soon as the mother resumes her care of him, and satisfies his hunger. Ecstatic experiences in later life have their roots in such reunions with the mother. A child that has an attitude of basic trust in the world will handle well stresses in later life. Insight into the genesis of the basic trust is of highest import for education. One need not fear to spoil an infant by too much affectionate attention. Later, when the child has learned to speak it will not be difficult to induce him to forego certain gratifications. The price paid for the little bit of training that can be achieved before the acquisition of language is too high. The child can bear frustrations only with great difficulty and at great expense to himself; his psychical apparatus is not yet sufficiently developed to tolerate frustration.

The sensitive erogenous zone changes with the child's advent into the anal phase of development. He experiences pleasurable sensations in connection with the processes of elimination, and develops curiosity and interest in his excrements. The attitude of the mother towards his excrements may be quite confusing for the child. He is praised for depositing his feces into the pot, but the same product is treated with disgust if placed outside of it. In addition the mother first admires the child's production, but then empties the pot and flushes the contents away.

For the small child his first experiences on the toilet seat can be very frightening. Accompanied by a mighty roar and rush of water his productions disappear into a dark abyss. The child is not at all certain that something similar and terrible will not happen to him as well. In the past, mothers were insistent on toilet training their children as early as possible. They took considerable pride in reporting their successes in this regard to their friends. As a rule today's children are brought up less rigidly. When the child is ready, he toilet trains himself, and the danger of creating a basis for a later character neurosis has been avoided. The excretory processes carry many conspicuous implications. To be unclean is disgusting, repellent, to be repellent is not decent, and people like to be considered decent and proper. The morality of the anal phase has primitive norms of cleanliness and decency. If the teaching of cleanliness is undertaken in an unreasonable manner, the growth of reaction formations is stimulated. The pleasure in smearing and messing is warded off and character traits of excessive preoccupation with cleanliness, propriety, and an anxious exactitude come into being. When children give up their desire to smear under undue pressure they often simultaneously lose their active striving in general, and with them their interest in the external world.

So far we have turned our attention only to the libidinal development. There are, however, other than libidinal drives. How we name this second kind of drive is not very significant, but we know that the desire for activity and the pleasure in activity and also aggressive behavior have their roots in this drive. To begin with, the infant is concerned with satisfactions of drives with a passive aim only, but as he gradually begins to move about, to indulge in some motor activity, he seeks to discover things and all this with evident pleasure. Later his inquisitiveness which gives him pleasure tempts him to make voyages of discovery which can be vexing for his parents. He collides with the furniture, pulls at bits of his own and others' clothing, turns over chairs, pulls the cat's tail, falls down and gets up again, pounds on the piano keys and so on. Along with his passive needs a striving towards vigorous activity is developing. We relate this activity to what is generally called the aggressive drive. I am reluctant to use this common expression. I believe that in using it we probably name not the drive but its infantile precursor. It would be more adequate to speak of a drive towards active mastery of the world, a drive towards self-realization. But we had better not belabor this confusion in terminology and continue to use the expression *aggressive drive.*

Important developmental changes take place during the anal phase. The child learns to control his sphincters and his motor activity, and acquires language, a most important accomplishment. Speech makes it possible for him to renounce direct gratification, and make do with mastery of the world by magical means. "Mama back" he says to himself repeatedly when put to bed, and murmuring "mama" he falls asleep. The words give him the feeling of the mother's presence. At first speech is an instrument of magic, later it becomes a means to overcome the same magic. The parents help the latter process along by telling him what the world is like, and by confronting him with reality. They help him to counterbalance his world of magic.

The way in which a child makes use of his experiences is of great importance for his later life. Strict training in cleanliness before the child fully understands what he is supposed to do is particularly frustrating, and frustration generates aggression. The anal-sadistic phase is frequently mentioned in that context, and indeed, at this time, the child's rage is easily provoked. It needs no emphasis that enemas and laxatives call forth intense feelings of helplessness in the child. He experiences such treatment as a violation of his body, a rape. Let us review more closely the object relationships of the child to his parents and other persons concerned with his training. During the oral phase the infant is completely dependent on his mother who provides his sustenance and other gratifications linked to her person. I have already pointed out that the young child gains pleasure from his activity and that understanding parents foster that activity. The child experiences profound feelings of satiation and gratification, but confronted with the powerful impulses which flood his inner self he is also subject to rage, anxiety and painful feelings of abandonment. All these emotions are very intense, and the child does not yet have a psychic structure capable of mastering these intense impulses and emotions.

Considerable changes take place during the anal phase. The child begins to develop individuality and attempts to carry through his own intentions and enforce his will. This period is sometimes described as the first adolescence. Lack of understanding on the part of the parents can lead to failure in his first attempts to develop individuality. Lack of understanding can lead to the development of obstinate attitudes which disturb adaptation in later life or result in symptom formation. Obstinacy affects the character formation unfavorably, it interferes with the development of genuine independence. Obstinacy is pliancy reversed. Genuine independence is the capacity to solve problems in a personal way and is a creative form of adaptation. One hears and reads references to the ambivalence of the child's relationship to his parents. Ambivalence means that the emotional relationship simultaneously contains love, affection, compassion and rage, anger, hostility and self-hatred.

The term ambivalence signifies little, unless we indicate what kind of ambivalence is meant. The child during the anal phase has an intensive emotional bond to his mother, and at the same times has a strong need for opposition. If the parents permit themselves to be drawn into a power struggle with their child, the need to oppose them can easily turn into stubbornness and obstinacy. As soon as the child becomes able to perceive his world and recognize its features, problems of jealousy occur. He would like to have his mother and father to himself, the birth of a sibling carries with it pleasure perhaps, but also many problems. The child's feelings in general, and particularly those rooted in the aggressive drive, are exceedingly passionate. The notion that children are angels; pure, affectionate, and without fault does not coincide with reality. The emotions of children are powerful and vehement, but they do not have the adults' capacities to deal with such emotions. That means that they urgently need the help of the parents in managing their feelings. If the parents do not deal competently with the problems of the anal phase, typical defense mechanisms make their appearance. A child who has experienced helplessness and a simultaneous lack of parental support in his predicament, acquires an inclination to treat others in the same way he felt he was treated. Children in the anal phase of development can be conspicuously cruel to animals and sadistic toward other children. They inflict on others what they experienced themselves. The child feels tormented by his parents when he is harshly forced to abide by their rules in regard to cleanliness and other activities. The transformation of passive sufferance into active behavior is one of the means to manage frustration and the aggressive feelings generated by it. The child also makes use of the defense mechanism of reversal into the opposite. He can become excessively clean and live in fear of soiling himself and others. A defense that is too intense results in developmental disturbances. The suppressed impulses fail to develop further to the next level, but remain unchanged. It is of course much better for the child to learn to manage his impulses than to repress them. It is easy to direct the child to substitute gratifications for the original pleasure in smearing. In this fashion we teach the child to make use of sublimation, i.e., to satisfy instinctual impulses with an activity which begins by being quite similar to the original instinctual aim, but in time can change into one equally satisfying yet quite remote from that aim.

The phallic phase follows upon the anal. We also call it the oedipal period, a designation appropriate primarily when we examine the phase from the viewpoint of the relationship of child and parents. Freud's ideas about this period of childhood called forth indignant opposition; people could not bear the thought that children experience intense, even violent emotions and impulses directed towards the parents. We must not lose ourselves in speculations about this theme, nor do we intend to adhere to a rigid model, but we shall describe what the child experiences during this period of his development. Before we discuss the oedipal phase I should like to add one more remark about jealousy. On entering the oedipal period the child has already learned to some extent to deal with this powerful emotion, because his intense needs always provide causes for jealous reactions. A new sibling in the family forces the child to deal with the task of sharing his parents' love with others. The manuever of the child's dealing with his jealous emotions will depend on many factors. It is of significance whether the intruding baby is a sister or a brother. Was the child prepared by the parents for the baby's arrival? It is a bitter experience for the child in the anal phase to observe that the mother produces so precious an object, while one's own productions are of fleeting value only and are flushed away. Present-day students no longer ask me whether children know that babies come out of the mother's body. Children observe the smallest changes in the mother's appearance. It is difficult to believe that there are still people who assume that children fail to notice the increasing girth of their fashionably thin mother.

We shall now turn to the changes which occur as the child enters the phallic phase. We shall begin with the development of the boy.

The transition from the anal to the phallic phase takes place by way of an intermediate phase which we call the urethral. It is impossible not to see that the little boy is very proud of his accomplishments in this regard. His mother has fostered that pride by praising him when he succeeded in urinating into the toilet bowl. We know that little boys greatly enjoy controlling this physiological function, and that quite often the urinating games engaged in by boys acquire a competitive character. A minor displacement of the gratification has occurred when the boy begins to play with the garden hose. Everyone knows how intense the pleasure is which the child derives from such activities.

The boy's attention is drawn to his penis, and his interest in it continues to become greater through the processes of maturation. He observes that he experiences erections, and that the manipulations of the penis provides him with pleasurable sensations. Parents who meet this development with anxiety and discomfort easily transfer these feelings to the child. Under such circumstances we observe little boys who get panic-stricken when they have an erection. It is then necessary to soothe their fears. What are the consequences of the feelings and sensations aroused in the child by his maturation processes on his relationship to the parents, or, to use our psychoanalytic terminology, on his object relationships? Let us recapitulate what we have learned about the development of instinctual life. During the early phases of development the infant was entirely dependent on the mother. In his relationship to her he experienced many kinds of pleasurable gratification. He was fondled, warmed, fed, and a longing for the satisfaction of these instinctual aims was always with him. We described them as passive instinctual aims. Pleasure in activity makes its appearance, and the mastery of the motoric functions, of the sphincters, and finally of speech adds to the awakening pleasure in discovery and enterprise. The passive needs do not disappear with the boy's entry into the phallic phase, but active strivings markedly predominate in that period. The little boy no longer wants to be treated as a baby, he wants to be mother's big boy, he assumes a chivalrous attitude towards her, and wants to be admired, thus displaying the forerunners of manly behavior. Libidinal sexual impulses are connected with this active attitude. The activity becomes intensified and acquires a different emphasis. We can state that a fusion of libidinal and aggressive impulses takes place. This theoretical idea aids us in understanding the phenomena which we observe at this stage. At times this fusion remains incomplete. We are familiar with men who are unable to assume an active role toward women, and are capable of sexual intercourse only when they assume a passive role. In summary we can say that in this phase the penis has become the primary erotogenic zone, and the little boy has assumed the posture of active conquest.

We turn now to object relationships. The formulations one encounters on reading descriptions of the oedipal relationship are often over simplified. It is said that the child has an active sexual attitude to his mother and hates his father. That is the meaning of the references that are made about the boy as a little Oedipus. Oedipus married his mother and slew his father. We must not forget that expressions like oedipal phase and Oedipus complex refer to particularly complicated and highly involved situations. We have already mentioned that passive and active impulses occur simultaneously. Similarly different feelings towards the mother are experienced at the same time. The boy has intense sexual curiosity about his mother's body, he wants to see it, to touch it and expresses his desire for much physical affection. But the attitude to the mother is not only positive; the mother cannot help but disappoint her little boy. She can only partially fulfill his wishes. He has to acknowledge that much as she loves her little son, her husband is the most important person in her life. He, the boy, sleeps alone in his room, while mother and father sleep together, and in the same bed. The little boy has to leave the bathroom during the mother's bath, but the father may remain with her. The boy hears sounds which indicate that activities between them take place from which he is excluded. Naturally, because of all of that, the boy is angry at his mother. We may speak of his ambivalent attitude toward the mother: This says little, unless we recognize clearly what the features of and motivations for this ambivalence are. We can learn much more about the oedipal child than about the infant, because he lets us know how he feels, and if he has been raised by understanding parents, he will himself tell us about his inner experiences. Accordingly, we can say that the little boy's feelings towards his mother are ambivalent. A strong positive striving is in danger of being disrupted because the son has to share his mother with someone else and feels disappointed. But what are the boy's feelings towards his father? It is not the view of psychoanalysis that he hates his father and wishes him to die. No, it is not at all as simple as that. On the contrary, the little boy loves his father. He enjoys their being together immensely—their excursions in the car, their playing, fishing, and engaging in many other common activities. The father knows so much, he can tell so many stories, he has many hobbies. Finally, his daily work is very important. How could the family get along without the father? The little boy is fully aware of the importance of the father's presence. He loves his father dearly, yet another set of feelings is also present in his mind. If the father were not to come home one day, he, the boy, would take care of mother. Perhaps not yet right away, but after a while, soon. The child's sense of time is as yet not well-developed, and he takes seriously the phrase his mother uses so frequently, "You are mother's big boy." Hence, here too, ambivalent feelings are in evidence, and the boy finds himself in a difficult emotional situation. Many and varied factors can evoke feelings of disappointment and hostility. The secret death wishes against the father can be kindled by a seemingly trivial cause, and the child under such circumstances experiences a profound internal conflict. He will most certainly react with the development of a feeling of guilt.

A specific form of anxiety adds itself to the problems which the boy struggles with in this period. This anxiety, to be discussed now, disturbs his emotional balance and has important consequences for his development. There are parents who because of their own anxieties or their neurotic attitudes react with threats to the boy's display of pride in his penis, as for instance when he wants to demonstrate to them the long arch which he can produce with his urinary stream. He is threatened with damage to his penis, even with its total loss, e.g., characters in stories who have lost a finger are held before him as examples of punishment meted out for forbidden activities. If the thumb can be cut off, why not also the penis? The little boy fears castration. He has in the meantime discovered that his mother or his little sister or playmate lacks the organ that he is so proud of. These observations contribute a second source to his castration anxiety. There is still a third factor to be considered. The little boy already had to learn to renounce some instinctual gratifications. He was deprived of the mother's breast, which was not part of his body, but which he considered as his property. In early infancy he could not distinguish mother's body from his own, just as he could not distinguish reality from the fantasies and images in his mind. In the anal phase he made the discovery that something which had been in his body emerged from it and fell off. If he was given an enema he felt robbed of something which palpably had been part of his body. He may have been subjected to a tonsillectomy, an operation which still is carried out much too frequently without regard to its psychic consequences. All this lends credence to the idea that he could be deprived of his penis. Obviously there are many different reasons to justify the boy's castration fears. If these become too pronounced the boy's development is disturbed. When the hostility to the father and the castration anxiety exceed the average intensity and the boy can no longer master his feelings and anxieties, the probability is great that he will remain fixated on this level of development and fail to mature into a psychologically mature man.

So far we have described the constellation known as the positive Oedipus complex. One also speaks of the negative Oedipus complex which is understood more fully in connection with the boy's total psychic development. We have already called attention to the fact that the boy directs passive instinctual strivings towards both parents. These are mainly gratified by the mother, but certainly also by the father. In wholesome family settings, the father encourages his son's active propensities. In authoritarian families, however, much is forbidden and little is encouraged. We have already remarked that the child readily develops guilt feelings; a threatening father will certainly evoke castration anxiety in his son. The little boy can become so burdened by anxiety and guilt that he relinquishes his positive oedipal attitude. He no longer acts the role of his mother's little knight, who, small though he is, enters the competition against his powerful father. Instead, he surrenders to the father and seeks gratification in passively receiving his father's love. The mother becomes his rival, and one speaks accurately of the boy's feminine identification. This can be clearly observed in the boy's behavior. The little boy shows signs of becoming effeminate. He develops an inclination to play with dolls, and to join the girls in their games. He will adjust his behavior to please others, since it is important for him to receive love, attention, and appreciation, and avoid competitive struggles. I have already pointed out that some of the foundations for jealousy of his mother were prepared in the anal phase. The mother can produce a baby, what he produces is quickly discarded. In the negative oedipal constellation the mother becomes the rival and the father the love object. In this constellation passive homosexuality has one of its origins. Regression to the anal phase takes place, and the stimulation of the anal area and the sensations related to it again become significant sources of pleasure. Accordingly, one can designate the negative Oedipus complex as homosexual and the positive as heterosexual. The bisexual attitude is an ever-present part of our psychic endowment. Every boy is interested in his father's sexual organs, and a sexual interest in one's own sex in the course of development is not pathological, unless the passive feminine attitude is strong enough to interfere with the advent of masculine attitudes. One can state that the negative Oedipus complex is always normally present. Only the excessive sexualization of the related emotions when used as a defense against the heterosexual attitude is pathological.

Very often a passive feminine attitude is influenced by the

boy's need to provoke punishment. When condemned by the punitive superego the passive-feminine attitude acquires a provocative air, to which the father reacts with punitive measures. He loses his temper, denounces the boy, and often attacks him bodily. In this fashion the child gains attention and concern, albeit in a negative form. He is at the same time an object of concern and punishment. We call such attitudes masochistic, and shall return later to the study of their significance. Some children who give the impression of aggressiveness and whose behavior is indeed difficult to bear are in fact masochistic. They crave punishment as a sign of concern and interest in them by the people around them. Their misbehavior is not the expression of a healthy aggressive drive and therefore it is tormenting and difficult to bear.

When the development is favorable, passive instinctual impulses directed toward one's own sex are subject to sublimation. Well-adapted forms of gratification of the passive needs come into being, for example, in the capacity to admire accomplishments of others, to accept graciously what one is offered, and to serve an ideal.

A child who has mastered the difficulties of the oedipal phase of development is temporarily free of instinctual problems. During the school years the developmental emphasis is mainly on the growth of the ego. The span of the child's world widens appreciably, and he discovers new potentialities in and outside of himself. The unfolding of these potentialities is aided and directed by a healthy ego ideal whose demands are capable of fulfillment: The ego should not be too inhibited by the commands and prohibitions of an excessively severe superego. The child's bonds to his mother help prepare a wholesome attitude towards the other sex. He has learned to fight his battles, and has identified with his father. He is capable of honest competition, guilt feelings and castration anxiety remain within tolerable limits and do not drive him into passivity. A child developing this way will direct his feelings to a heterosexual object in adolescence. But before we turn to adolescence we shall explore the corresponding female development.

The oedipal phase of the girl, like that of the boy, is determined by her experiences in the preceding phases of development. One often hears the question: Is the cause of the neurosis to be found in the oedipal or pre-oedipal phase? The answer of necessity must be that the unresolved difficulties of the total childhood development are responsible for the damage done to the unfolding of the personality. The way in which the child progresses through the oedipal period is co-determined by everything that preceded it. It is of great importance whether the parents demonstrated to the little girl that they are happy about having a daughter.

We emphatically contradict the view that awareness of one's own sex and of the difference between the sexes does not occur until the oedipal phase. The observer of young children is immediately struck by the different and typical behavior patterns of little boys and girls. The oedipal phase involves a definitive step in sexual development, and identification with one's own sex, and the process of becoming familiar with the experience of being a man or a woman. Biological maturation awakens an increased curiosity about the sexual organs and here the little girl makes a painful discovery. She discovers the anatomical differences of the sexes. She can react in various ways to this discovery, but a feeling of disappointment is always a part of her reaction. She makes the mother responsible for her disappointment. The mother, after all, plays the most important role in her life. The psychoanalytic theory of the female development is sometimes met with indignation, or with ridicule, and the theory is dismissed as nothing but a fantasy of the psychiatrist. However, one can also hear an occasional voice remarking that the speaker had observed his own little girl in an attempt to urinate standing up, and she was quite sad about her failure to perform this function like her little brother. The little girl is unquestionably fascinated by her brother's ability in that regard, and by the organ that enables him to perform in this fashion. A female student reported an interesting observation: She had seen her little daughter look with interest and some concern at the neighbor's little boy urinating in the street. In the following night she awoke crying from a dream: "Mummy I had a watering can, a pretty watering can, and when I tried to water the flowers, it did not work. It was broken." The mother explained to her that she was not "broken," comforted her and assured her that father and mother were delighted with their little daughter. A day later the mother heard the child sing to herself over and over a "poem" she had made up: "We don't have it, we don't get it, we stay as we are."

The discussion of this subject may have tempted one to assume a humorous and cheerful view of the girl's problem, but if the parents fail to help their child to overcome such difficulties the results are all but cheerful. The future development of the little girl can suffer. When we deal with the psychopathology of specific disorders we shall see what symptom-formations and detrimental character deviations are caused by the female castration complex.

Every girl will deal in her own way with the disappointment, the anger at the mother, and jealousy of the supposedly better equipped male generated in this developmental phase. The child's responses are determined by the situation in which she finds herself, and the parents play the main role in shaping this situation. The disappointment with the mother is an important factor in the intensification of the attachment to the father. The father's manhood is a source of the little girl's particular attraction to him in the phallic phase. She enters into the oedipal phase in a manner much like the little boy. She loves her mother, but the latter is at the same time her rival. She is fascinated by her father but also disappointed in him. If the father rejects his little daughter's aspirations to be his "wife" too roughly or if the mother's attitude burdens her with unbearable guilt feelings, the possibility is greater that the negative Oedipus complex will become dominant and will influence the girl's further development. The child may stubbornly refuse to relinquish the fantasy that one day she will receive or grow a penis like the boy. She regresses to a relationship with the mother which prevailed in the pre-oedipal phase, she gives up her interest in the father and represses it. As in the boy we mostly observe both forms of the Oedipus complex simultaneously. As in the boy's case, excessive guilt feelings and the castration complex will interfere with the girl's acceptance of her female sexual role. If the development proceeds on a healthy course the child will be able to successfully enter that role and the state of maturity as an adult. The negative Oedipus complex interferes with the man's development, the penis envy with that of the woman. At the same time a tendency towards regression becomes manifest. The child, unable to master the oedipal problems, escapes into the infantile position. A normal development of the little girl leads to an identification with the mother. The little girl playing with her dolls is in fantasy a little mother. In the woman's emotional life the father is later replaced by the husband. The relationship to her father retains considerable significance in the healthy woman's conscious experience. When she succeeds in accepting her own femininity the relationship to the mother retains a warm and affectionate quality, unencumbered by the early tensions between them. One of the neurotic woman's characteristics is her abiding hostility to the mother which may be open or hidden. Objectively the much-hated mother is usually no worse than many other mothers, but the infantile jealous rage and the bitter anger about having received less than one's due in such cases have remained unchanged and in full force. Freud has pointed out that the husband sometimes becomes heir to the hostility towards the mother instead of the love for the father, a circumstance which does not favor the chances of success in marriage.

A wholesome sexual relationship can provide for a woman a valuable compensation for the disappointments of her youth. In a relationship with a man who is neither too demanding nor too stinting with his affection and is considerate of her needs, she will experience his sexual organ as something that is their common possession, and when a child arrives the persistent early wish of the little girl will find its fulfillment in it. This development is not always optimally successful. When, however, sufficient adaptability is available the scars of the early injuries do not hinder happiness in later life. The decisive issue is dependent on quantitative relationships and intensities in the interplay of psychic forces, in which the object relationships play a significant role. They often determine whether, in a given situation, a healthy adaptation or a neurotic reaction results.

After the oedipal period follows the latency period during which the instinctual tensions are quiescent. This period is relatively free of instinctual problems. Normally the Oedipus complex has had a more or less complete resolution—the psychic energy bound up in it becomes available for the growth of the ego, the child's world expands, and the child makes use of his potential. The new discoveries are charged with much emotion, the mutual relationships with schoolmates gain in depth and differentiation. The manifestations of a neurotic development at this stage are listlessness, lack of initiative, conflict with authorites, an inclination to isolation and excessive sexual preoccupation. Repressed rage expresses itself in nail biting, headaches, and other psychosomatic complaints. Bed wetting is evidence of much castration anxiety and of frustrated fantasies of omnipotence.

We have described in the foregoing the Oedipus complex of the boy and the girl and have attempted to illuminate the child's inner experiences. For didactic purposes we shall follow this up with a more schematic presentation.

The boy's Oedipus complex contains erotic attitudes to the mother which result in disappointment, and admiration of the father which is coupled with jealousy. The negative Oedipus complex is based on a passive-feminine attitude to the father, and the simultaneous experience of the mother as one's rival. When this constellation is particularly intense, the negative Oedipus complex acquires a strongly sexualized or masochistic character, thereby incurring pathological significance. In this process castration anxiety is of decisive importance. The pathological elaboration of the negative Oedipus complex and its roots in the castration anxiety has great significance for the genesis of neurosis in the male.

The castration complex is significant for the girl in the form of penis envy. She too experiences both the positive and negative Oedipus complex. The girl's intense bond to the mother is often disturbed by her discovery of the anatomical difference between the sexes. She turns to the father with her emotional needs. If the formation of the positive Oedipus complex miscarries she falls back upon the relationship to the mother and gets into rivalry with the father. The negative Oedipus complex has in that case gained the upper hand. In the formation of neuroses penis envy plays the same role for the woman as the passive feminine position does for the man. Unconsciously she is no more able to give up the wish to have a penis than the man is able to give up his sublimated passive wishes.

While examining the female development we must not forget that the girl has to choose as an object of her love a person whose sex differs from that of her original love object. She has to learn to direct to the father the wishes which she initially directed to the nursing mother. The little boy remains faithful to the mother, his original object, but he must alter his attitude to her. He has to develop an active, conquering attitude instead of the original passive attitude.

The simple statement that the man is active, the woman passive is not correct if stated without the required qualification. The woman must also be capable of active mastery. The way to the latter is through the identification with the mother. The sublimation of the woman's masculine inclinations also contributes to her mastery of the problems of maturation. The normally developing male will sublimate his passive feminine strivings; his heterosexual passive needs can be gratified in his love life. Developmental processes continue as long as the person's psyche has not become entirely rigid, but adolescence is the stage in which a person's character acquires its definitive form. We observe a recrudescence of the oedipal problems, and a second stage of the sexual development takes place. At this time masturbation is the main problem. The struggle against it will be the more troublesome the less tolerant the superego has become. Again the development takes place in constant interaction with the young person's environment. Undue severity of the parents will make this development more difficult and painful, their candor and understanding acceptance of the natural course of sexual maturation will favor a normal development.

A very severe superego initiates depressive reactions; sometimes the conflict ends in the asceticism of puberty, so clearly described by Anna Freud: The ego ideal of the ascetic proclaims the renunciation of all instinctual gratification; the most stern prohibitions are understandably connected with this demand. When the fears of punishment are very intense, a hypochondriacal preoccupation with ruminations about venereal disease may result. Self-condemnatory attitudes can be projected and give impetus to paranoid elaborations. Sometimes the stern morality causes feelings of deep discouragement, the feeling that one really is a very bad person. Serious psychic pathology can result in consequence of such feelings. The person does not succeed in establishing a heterosexual position in fantasy and in reality will be inclined toward homosexuality. In adolescence this inclincation can still be overcome.

Against the dark background sketched above, the normal adolescent development provides a picture of shining contrast. Healthy young people discover the world and themselves, and their difficulties and conflicts are those unavoidable tensions in life which can be termed normal. Difficulties and challenges stimulate the growth and maturation of a normal child. Being mostly conscious these challenges are capable of optimal management.

One has the impression that youth today has a tendency to heterosexual experimentation and a need to try many different experiences in sexual life. Many of these experiments are stimulated by curiosity, the wish to challenge the prevailing norms and the fear of masturbation. We cannot as yet state what consequences the altered patterns of sexual behavior have had or will have for the psychic development.

During adolescence boys and girls get acquainted with each other. They undergo processes of identification which will later determine their vocational choices. A neurotic development inhibits the ability to make such a choice, and distorts it owing to conscious and unconscious needs to oppose or contradict environmental influences.

Interest in hobbies begins to develop; they complement the gratifications stemming from work, and, in view of the increasingly available time for leisure in our society, they grow in importance for the satisfactory functioning of the personality. Healthy aggression can be gratified through interest in political issues. We commonly find a strong preoccupation with religion in adolescence, which, though sometimes based on neurotic conflict, at other times is the expression of the adolescent's quest for cause and meaning of all things involving him. Only adherents of a narrow-minded and outdated rationalistic view will discourage the adolescent's thoughts about religion and his searching for the meaning of existence. These are, along with his sexual emotions the most important experiences of the adolescent. The healthy person prepares through adolescence to take the step into adulthood. The neurotically predisposed lack inner freedom, the defense mechanisms have caused character deformations, and their characterological armor impedes all relationships with the world.

Communication between the different agencies of the personality is hindered; anxiety and depression are always in the background. There is considerable probability that pressures of life, the unavoidable disappointments at work and in marriage will precipitate the development of a flourishing neurosis. In the chapters dealing with the individual neuroses we shall discuss these matters in detail. Our insight into the experimental world of neurotic people enables us to help them, and in future our knowledge should enable us to devise preventive measures.

THE FOUNDATIONS OF PSYCHOANALYTIC THEORY

Before we proceed to the problems of the individual neuroses, we shall review briefly the structure of psychoanalytic theory. We have made use of this theory in the preceding chapters, and shall now deal with it in a more exact manner.

The distinction conscious-unconscious is the subject of the topographical point of view. We visualize the conscious and the unconscious as realms of the psyche. We can regard the same concepts, conscious and unconscious, in a functional sense, as qualities of psychic processes. This last view is the one increasingly preferred by psychoanalysts. We utilize the structural viewpoint when our attention is mainly directed to the id, ego, superego and ego ideal as elements of personality structure. Some psychoanalysts consider the ego ideal a function of the superego. These two aspects of the superego are, however, always distinct from one another. It is therefore proper to speak of the ego ideal when one wishes to delineate their differences. The ego has at its disposal the cognitive function, reality testing, and the defense mechanisms. The ego can ward off the drive, but it also can master instinctual impulses through sublimation. Considering the energy of the drive one can also state that the ego neutralizes the drive energy. We have already discussed the id when we introduced the concepts of the libido and aggression as denoting the two basic drives.

Structures have meaning only in connection with functions. This is the place to mention the third viewpoint of the theory, the dynamic aspect of the interplay of forces within the personality. These forces can have various quantitative relationships, they are of different intensities. In examining these we apply the economic viewpoint, which is concerned with the relative power of drive and defense, and with the intensity of the feelings and actions as they derive respectively from desire and defense. When we examine all these phenomena from the developmental aspect we apply the genetic viewpoint of the psychoanalytic theory. Instinctual impulses and the manner in which they are dealt with by ego, superego, and ego ideal have biological significance for adaptation. The attention given to these problems represents the adaptive point of view of the theory. Man adapts to the social situation, to society. Erikson (1950) has comprehensively discussed this viewpoint in his book, *Childhood and Society*, which already has become part of the classical psychoanalytic literature. Society, its educational principles, and the intrapsychic structure with its dynamics must be brought in relation to each other. Only then can they be properly understood.

Mothers rear their children so that they will fit into and assert themselves in a given society, and the society prescribes the educational principles. Awareness of these connections could contribute much towards the overcoming of irrational child-rearing measures and irrational patterns of society. Adaptation is more than a passive adjustment to circumstances, adaptation implies also an active altering of his environment by man to suit his needs.

The points of view mentioned above and their mutual interrelationships are represented by the psychoanalytic metapsychology. The emphasis is on the prefix meta in so far as the metapsychology seeks to bridge the gap between psychology and biology; but the different viewpoints also have a purely psychological meaning; as a heuristic principle metapsychology gives us excellent service. In examining a psychic phenomenon we seek to evaluate it in terms of adaptation of the superego's demands and ego ideal expectations; we inquire into its defense aspects, and question which instinctual needs are gratified, and what its significance is for the person's self esteem, i.e., its narcissistic value.

I should like to illustrate this once more with an example: Depression is a disturbance of adaptation. In looking at it in terms of the drive, we find frustrated passive strivings and a turning of the aggression against the self. Secondarily the depressed person directs his aggression against others as well; his distressed mien, his sadness and gloom, make it impossible for them to enjoy a pleasurable life. The depressed person's superego is too severe and too powerful, his ego ideal too exalted. Depressive people often have unconscious fantasies of grandeur. As we turn to the depressed person's ego we observe a preponderance of defense, a disturbance of the cognitive function and of all activity, and inhibition of motor expression. We ask how did all this come into being and thereby apply the genetic approach. We shall discuss this in detail in the framework of our study of the specific neurosis.

These comments make it clear that a psychic phenomenon can be fully understood only if we apply all approaches we have mentioned in our study. I should like therefore to repeat the formulation made previously: metapsychology intends to build a bridge between biology and psychology. Metapsychology is an important heuristic principle. It seems important to me to point out again that the meaning of a character formation, of neurotic behavior, or of a neurotic symptom becomes clear only when we have examined the respective phenomenon utilizing the topographic, the structural, economic and genetic-dynamic approaches, when we have examined what effect all this has on the adaptation, and finally, when we investigate the connections of the respective psychic event with narcissim, libido and aggression.

After this introduction we are sufficiently prepared to turn to the problems of the pathology of specific neuroses.

2

THEORY OF THE NEUROSES[1]

THE CONCEPT neurosis includes many manifestations which result from a conflict between the ego and the repressed instinctual impulses. There occur somatic complaints, as expression of psychic tensions and disharmonies in the personality, difficulties in interpersonal relationships, particularly in the sexual sphere, and multiple learning and working inhibitions. In no other area of psychiatry do the signs of crisis in our science appear as evident as in the theory of the psychopathology of the neuroses.

NOSOLOGICAL CONSIDERATIONS

One frequently hears the objection that it is impossible to devise a diagnostic classification of the neuroses analogous to Kraepelin's classification of the psychoses and, if one were to be devised, it would be worthless. The argument goes: What does the diagnosis communicate to us? It provides us with a name, a tag, but it does not advance our knowledge. Objec-

[1] I wish to thank all those who collaborated with me in writing this chapter: Dr. J. Lampl-de Groot reviewed the text and made a number of suggestions which I have followed up to advantage; my colleagues at my hospital, Drs. J. Bastiaans, G. A. Ladee, J. H. Thiel and N. Treurniet, worked with me on extensive portions of the text. The division into hysterical neuroses and those related to hysteria was worked out in collaboration with them. Their experience as teachers was most helpful in planning this book.

tions against nosology in general, and particularly against the Kraepelinian system carry some weight in psychiatry, and are virtually inescapable in the realm of the neuroses. Here the transitions are so fluid and gradual that one doubts the advantage of thinking in terms of disease entities. In addition neurotic conditions can change into psychotic disorders, and the borderline between reasonably adapted behavior and neurotic behavior is also mobile and fluctuating. It appears not very fruitful to include a third class of disorders of the mind between neuroses and psychoses; difficulties would multiply since one would have to define more borders between them. Those who believe that one should discard the Kraepelinian system approach all nosology with scepticism. Among them are many who adhere to a genetic-dynamic view of the neuroses. Their argument can be put approximately into sentences like the following: "Describe what you see before you, what processes take place, what tensions are created by the unsatisfactory use of defense mechanisms; but classificatory statements are of little interest for us." The division of the neuroses and their classifications must be subjected to a close study. To orient ourselves, we shall use the following points of reference: (1) classification and the problem of the fluctuating transitions; (2) the limited number of possible diagnoses; (3) the collection of data versus diagnostics; (4) clinical-diagnostic versus the genetic-dynamic approach.

Classification and the problem of fluctuating transitions. An argument that is often brought up against classification is the easy overlapping between different neurotic conditions. Many patients suffering from a hysterical neurosis also have obsessive traits and are subject to neurotic depression. If our nosological system shows that more cases fall outside than inside of certain categories, we ask if such a system is at all useful? The existence of transitional states between certain categories is in itself no reason to dispense with all classification. If we can state how many features of one disorder and how many of another a patient shows, we have supplied as much information about him as we do by placing him into a specific diagnostic group, provided we do not treat the diagnoses as almost metaphysical entities. In his study of psychopathy and neuroses, Carp (1947) has pointed out that fluctuating transitions are not the definitive argument against a classification which is based on discernible differences. Edmund Burke has formulated the same opinion thus, "Though now man can draw a stroke between the confines of night and day, yet light and darkness are upon the whole tolerably distinguishable."

The limited number of possible diagnoses. Another objection to classification claims that the number of diagnostic entities is too small for a proper nosology. Where shall we place the work inhibitions which bring many patients to the social worker, the psychologist and psychiatrist? Where do those patients belong who seek help because they are troubled by homosexual fantasies and dreams? They do not fit into the customary diagnostic classification, but is that a reason to do away with diagnostic criteria altogether? I believe rather that we have reason to expand our nosological system. Disease manifestations change, they are not rigid entities; they change with the social and cultural situation of which they often are but one expression. The fainting of young girls was once normal, a little bit of hysteria was part of the mental endowment of the young woman of the better classes. Today warding off of the affect is the common pattern, and the lovers "play it cool." The grand hysteria, the major hysterical attack has become a rarity, but other neurotic conditions have become very common among girls who have such a miserable time with themselves and the world. One can no longer term these conditions hysterical, one has to set up new terms for new conditions. Indeed Abraham (1920) has done this in a work that justly has become famous. We shall discuss it later in detail.

The collection of as much data as possible versus diagnostics. A further argument against nosology is as follows: Of what use is it if we call someone an obsessive-compulsive neurotic? We have to know a great deal more about him. We must assemble as much data about him as possible before we can understand him and we must make use of all possible points of view—psychological, sociological, ethological and biochemical—in our diagnosis. In my opinion such an argument offers too much extraneous material. What should we begin to do with all the collected data? Would a film covering the whole life of our patient bring us closer to our aim? One would soon discover that this comprehensive material would be of little use. What we gain in factual material acquires meaning only when we arrange it into a definite frame of reference. Only what is relevant in understanding and helping the patient is serviceable material. Our aim is insight and not a mass of material. We gain insight by bringing concepts, theories and hypotheses in relation to the material, and that implies judicious selection. Goethe's frequently cited sentence is worthy of note: "Das Höchste wäre: zu begreifen, dass alles Faktische schon Theorie ist." [2]

Anything that fails to facilitate our insight into the patient's suffering so that we may help him is irrelevant in the therapeutic situation. It is superfluous and often confusing. One has to ask the right questions but this is not all. When we have termed a patient a compulsive neurotic, we must not pretend that this is sufficient information about him; however, this diagnosis can be more significant than a mass of ill-assorted facts assembled by psychologists, sociologists, social workers, and biochemists. Representatives of auxiliary sciences of psychiatry can contribute something meaningful only when they reply to the clinician's questions. This applies

---

[2] This sentence defies translation. Its sense is that it is most desirable to comprehend that intelligent observation of facts implies and reveals the relevant theoretical framework.

to clinical work as well as to scientific research. Amassing of facts as such has nothing to do with knowledge. To view a diagnosis as an inadequate substitute for the demand that we "know everything," and to refuse to make a diagnosis because of such a view is a misconception of the theory of cognition.

Clinical-diagnostic versus genetic-dynamic approach. Psychoanalysts also raise objections against nosology. They point to the fact that so many patients have both hysterical and compulsive as well as other neurotic features, and that one knows little about a patient even after one has attached a diagnostic label to him. They maintain the significant issue is in the processes and in the interplay of forces which are at the root of the symptoms. It is difficult to argue against these objections. If one can do no more than supply labels one returns to the point at which Freud started. The diagnoses of hysteria and compulsive neurosis were common at the time Freud showed us what goes on inside the patients, which unconscious motivations lead to their disturbed adaptations. These subjects are of great interest to us. We do want to know what the dynamics are, which defense mechanisms the patient uses, how his superego and ego ideal function, whether his ego strength is sufficient, what course the development of his instinctual life has taken, and much more.

But does our interest in these questions and our conviction of the indispensability of the investigation of the dynamics and genetics imply that a precise description of the patient and the definition of specific forms of the neuroses, of neurotic syndromes, is without value and an anachronism? Certainly not! The descriptive psychological outline—a method which since the appearance of Jasper's *General Psychopathology* carries the unfortunate name of phenomenology, is always the first step in diagnosis. Every case history has to begin with a description. It is self-evident that this description is based on a certain point of view, but there is considerable difference between an immediate theoretical conclusion based on what the patient says, and the attempt to render as much as possible of what he tells us about his inner experiences in his own words. Descriptive and genetic-dynamic psychology are not mutually exclusive. No more is there a contradiction between the genetic-dynamic view, the exploration of the interplay of forces in the personality and the significance of the patient's life history on one side, and the nosological approach, the application of a division into neurotic syndromes on the other. On closer examination the arguments against thinking in terms of nosology appear spurious. The person who believes that he has completed his diagnostic work after finding a slogan, a magic formula, as it were, must certainly be emphatically refuted. But what compels us to misuse diagnostic classification in this manner? When one conceives of diagnostics in the broad sense of description of the symptoms, a definition of the syndrome and enumeration of the etiological factors leading to the disease, one cannot do without naming the appropriate syndrome, and just as certainly one cannot limit oneself to a mere diagnostic label. Disease entities in the original Kraepelinian sense, namely with a precisely defined cause, course, end-result and a pathological anatomical substratum do not exist, that much is certain. However, the conditions delineated by Kraepelin can be used as descriptively circumscribing the syndromes, and in that sense many of them are not only serviceable but indispensable. Kroll (1929) has pointed out that what impresses us frequently as "disease" is not the disease, but only a syndrome, called forth by different conditions, different constellations of varying factors and the joining together of some of these factors.

As such, nosological considerations need not be outdated because an old conception of disease entities proved impractical. I believe that incompetence—the inclination to theorize too rapidly, and insufficient skill in clinical diagnosis—also contributes to the rejection of the nosology founded by Kraepelin. One condemns what one fails to master. Endless assembling of factual data can also have the purpose of postponing the necessity of making a diagnosis. The concept of a single psychosis covering all mental illness is gratefully accepted when one lacks differentiating capacity. To act as if all previous efforts towards the establishment of a nosology were unnecessary signifies a want of thought and imagination.

At the end of these deliberations I should like to repeat once more what I mean by diagnosis. A good diagnosis consists of: (1) A description of the symptoms. (2) A definition of the disease syndrome in the sense of common combinations of symptoms, some of which may be more significant than others. (3) The investigation of the dynamics involved in the symptoms. And finally, (4) The exploration of the etiology, i.e., the psychogenic, constitutional, and organic factors, and of the influences of the close and extended environment. This is a form of diagnosis, which belongs to an integrated therapeutic science, to use an excellent term coined by Querido. It describes a method in which man is viewed within the different areas of his existence.

In the following pages I shall treat the theory of the neuroses from this position, and shall pay particular attention to the dynamic and genetic aspects of the theory.

MANIFESTATIONS OF THE NEUROSES

It is not astonishing that the neurotic symptoms and not the neurotic character are first to command our attention. The patient suffers from his symptoms, which provide his motive for turning to the physician. The psychiatrist diagnoses the neurotic character along with the symptoms. Historically the sequence was the same; the symptoms were investigated first, and then the neurotic character. The patient perceives his symptoms, senses that something alien is happening to him, and experiences a narrowing of his subjective freedom because of anxiety, conversion symptoms, or a disturbance of his work capacity. The symptom is rightly described as ego-alien. It is something which is experienced by the patient as not belonging to his self. In contrast to this his character is felt to be ego-syntonic, though the people close to the patient may occasionally wish that he had a different character.

The hysterical patient for example, suffers from nausea and difficulties of swallowing but perceives nothing unusual in her infantile manner of relating to others only as suppliers of her needs or as admirers. That is her concept of love. She says, "That's how I am," and takes herself for granted. Most people react differently to another person's symptoms than to his neurotic character. As a rule they feel compassion for the former and are irritated or constrained by the latter. Their own inner problems account in part for the difference in reaction.

We must differentiate between neurotic symptom and neurotic character in order to understand the psychopathology of the neuroses. W. Reich called particular attention to the neurotic character. His book on "Characteranalysis" is considered by many, myself among them, as one of the most significant psychoanalytic contributions. Reich rightly spoke of a character armor. The character of some persons has a defensive function. It serves to ward off drive, guilt feelings and anxiety. The consequence of this function of the character is impairment of psychic mobility. This is most clearly evident in the case of compulsive characters, concerned as they are with their principles and exaggerated scruples. The "armor" has the task of providing the person with a feeling of security, but in fact it sharply limits his freedom of movement.

Later on, the attention of the researchers was drawn to the

neurotic relationships and neurotic mental maneuvers. A neurotic relationship is undertaken for the unconscious purpose of reliving in it a neurotic conflict. The person "acts it out." Stated differently, the neurotic relationship represents an expression of the neurosis on the level of interpersonal relationships. Freud (1912) called attention to neurotic relationships in his eassy "On the Universal Tendency to Debasement in the Sphere of Love," and in other works. Many men find it impossible to have sexual relations with a woman toward whom they experience tender and friendly emotions— passion, tenderness and friendship has not been integrated into a unity. People with such difficulties have sexual relationships which remain unsatisfactory on the intimate personal level. They cannot experience love and desire at the same time; their relationships are neurotic.

We shall take our second example from the area of conflict with authority. Patients with such conflicts react adversely to their domineering superiors. They live out their conflict in the real situation, they establish a neurotic relationship with people in authority and in such situations are unable to act reasonably. They also manage to irritate even those not in authority, so that the latter become aggressive and display their less agreeable traits. The motives of this ill-adapted behavior are of course entirely unconscious. The patient forces others into a behavior pattern, into a role, which fits in with the patient's conflicts with authority. Such unconscious behavior patterns we designate as neurotic maneuvers. Frequently such maneuvers extend over long periods of time, they require time for their full development. An example: A woman who intensely but unconsciously envies all men falls passionately in love with a married man, who is well known for his faithfulness to his wife. She succeeds in gaining his love; he decides to separate from his wife and children and to marry her. At this moment she becomes infatuated with another man and rejects the man whose marriage she has destroyed. Her reaction is unmistakably triumphant. Behavior like hers we call a neurotic maneuver. The woman discharged her hostility, her hatred of men, which was rooted in her envy of them. The first passionate infatuation, the frenzied character of her feelings, the new involvement at the moment of conquest, all this is part of the neurotic maneuver. When intense sadomasochistic impulses participate in motivating the neurotic maneuver the situation can lead to tragedy. Suicide and homicide can occur as a result of the unmanageable jealousy of one of the partners.

To recapitulate: we can distinguish neurotic symptoms, neurotic characters, neurotic relationships and neurotic maneuvers. The neurosis can manifest itself in all or some of the forms mentioned above.

Unconscious jealousy and discontent with the feminine role can manifest itself in: (1) symptoms, like depression and deficient performance; (2) character traits, like artificiality; (3) neurotic relationships, like promiscuous behavior; and (4) in neurotic maneuvers. The knowledge of all these is indispensable for the understanding of the psychopathology of the relationships between the sexes.

Bergler (1946) in his book *Unhappy Marriage and Divorce*, compares the behavior of the neurotic with that of a man who plays many different records, but hears only the same melody. It is indeed striking that all his relationships bring nothing new, not even variations on the theme, but only repetitions of the same melody. In a non-neurotic relationship new facets constantly develop, the partners discover new possibilities in themselves, the scope of their common experiences unfolds and yet they remain true to themselves.

The diagnosis of a neurosis is insufficient if it limits itself to the symptoms and character traits, it must include the evaluation of the neurotic relationships and the neurotic maneuvers. The relationships to people in the environment are often the mirror image of the intrapsychic relations. Conscience and ego have their relations reflected in conflicts with authority, ego and id in the relations exclusively concerned with the gratification of sexual needs. I believe that certain maneuvers are as characteristic of neurotic conditions as the symptoms or character traits. We shall return to this idea in the next chapter.

One can limit the diagnostic description of a neurosis to the dynamic and genetic factors. When we spoke in favor of retaining a nosology with its definitions of types and syndromes we did not do it out of consideration for those who are unfamiliar with psychoanalytic categories, but because of the conviction that it is useful to be familiar with certain combinations of symptoms. I am certain that these combinations represent not only theoretically possible types but many that indeed occur in life and claim our attention again and again.

Carp (1947) has written about such types in the work already cited, for instance the hysterical swindler, the slanderer and others. On reading his descriptions one meets easily recognizable people. Having learned to recognize these typical people, the student, the psychiatrist in training, the psychologist or social worker is impelled to search for the unconscious motives for their behavior, and arrives at a consideration of the area of dynamic and genetic diagnosis. It is certainly useful to consider clinical pictures in the delineation of the neurosis from psychopathy and psychosis. I shall now make a few remarks about this topic. First, we shall take up the differences between neurosis and psychopathy and I shall then connect this with some observations about their relation to the psychoses and perversions.

PSYCHOPATHY—NEUROSIS—PSYCHOSIS—PERVERSION

Let us first decide what we mean by the term psychopathy. Because of their disharmonious personalities and abnormal behavior, psychopathic patients often become involved in serious conflicts with their environment. They emphatically ascribe the responsibility for their miseries to the environment. I shall not conceal the fact that I have often doubted the value of the concept of psychopathy. Psychopathic behavior can invariably be viewed as a consequence of neurotic conflicts and faulty development. However, one sees conditions in clinical experience for which the diagnosis of neurosis may be inexact. I shall offer some tentative conclusions, questions and propositions, and shall lay particular emphasis on some terminological clarification. Again and again one is disappointed by the conspicuous waste of time spent on discussion and argument before the relevant concepts have been delineated. If one omits preliminary agreement on terms and concepts, the conversation turns into a purely rhetorical exercise, without relation to clinical reality.

(a) The concept of psychopathy causes the most confusion. This occurs when the characteristic pattern, the main manifestations of which are dissocial behavior, an impoverishment of affect, is considered with a certain preconceived notion about its etiology, namely, that psychopathy is entirely based on innate constitutional factors. This notion is often connected with an open or secret therapeutic nihilism, and not infrequently also with the expression of hostile sentiments towards such patients. It is expressed in the phrase: "This good-for-nothing is never going to change." The inclination to ascribe a set of disease manifestations to a definite single cause is a tiresome heritage from the days of Kraepelin. Along with the disparagement of psychogenic factors this heritage has impeded the development of our understanding of the psychopathic patient. To think of psychopathy as exclusively caused by organic factors is unprofitable. In light of such thinking every neurotic in whom one may suspect the presence of constitutional disturbances becomes a psychopath. It is wasted effort just to move a patient from one category to another.

(b) The work of researchers interested in genetic issues, as for instance, Bowlby, Anna Freud, Hart de Ruyter, and others has proven that psychopathy can result from neglect in early infancy. Social and psychogenic factors must not be underestimated. Lampl-de Groot (1928) has called attention to the fact that certain milieu-generated conscious conflicts play a large role in the psychic life of psychopathic patients. These findings refute the "single cause" theory that psychopathy is an innate disturbance. One can also use the term psychopathy to describe a behavior pattern, rather than a disease entity. K. Eissler (1949) utilized Freud's differentiation in auto- and alloplastic reactions in separating neurosis from psychopathy. The neurotic primarily suffers himself, the psychopath primarily inflicts suffering on others. Some examples: A man given to neurotically motivated infidelity fully knows that he is unable to bind himself to one woman. He gives up all approaches to women and bears the distress of his loneliness.

A second patient enjoys many conquests, evokes many expectations, but attaches himself to no one permanently. When asked to justify his behavior, he will say, "One mustn't take these things too seriously, every woman enjoys a fling now and then." A third man, also subject to neurotic infidelity, enters into many love relationships; indeed he makes attempts to have them endure, but only to escape and disappoint his partners. He suffers more anguish than they, yet he is compelled to fail them again and again. The first patient is undoubtedly neurotic, the second psychopathic, the third occupies an intermediate position; he shows both auto- and alloplastic reactions. The following question comes to mind: Does not the second patient in spite of his alloplastic reaction suffer from his faithlessness, does he not conceal feelings of guilt under his frivolous remark? And does not the inhibited neurotic of our first example inflict suffering by his inability to love? Does he not deprive a woman longing for love of her chance to find a man? Is it not true that every inhibition, every autoplastic reaction also causes suffering for the environment? Do psychopathic persons indeed suffer less pain than neurotics? The happy-go-lucky, frivolous psychopathic scamp is more often the product of the imagination of a somewhat inhibited psychiatrist than a true diagnostic entity. It appears that there is only a relative difference between many alloplastic and autoplastic reactions. This quantitative variance does not mean that there are no distinctions between them. The aggressive impulses of the psychopathic patients are openly directed against the environmental figures, whereas the distress suffered by the environment of neurotic patients is more in the nature of a by-product. Since the neurotic person's ego ideal is quite different than that of the psychopath, he cannot express his impulses by direct action. The difference between auto- and alloplastic reactions can be frequently demonstrated; one has to bear in mind the fact that the pain which the neurotic patient inflicts on his environment is a secondary phenomenon, neither consciously nor even unconsciously intended by the patient.

In the course of my professional life I have become acquainted with most, perhaps with all interpretations of psychopathy. I followed the authorities and had faith in the old concepts of psychopathy. Later on I was very much impressed by the juxtaposition of autoplastic and alloplastic reactions. Later I was inclined to interpret all asocial manifestations as neurotic. I shall spare the reader further autobiographical details, and limit myself to the description of my current views.

All autoplastic reactions may be related to each other, neuroses and psychopathy may have much in common. Nevertheless, a person who lives out his conflicts in reality, i.e., acts out without restraint, and has a defective ego and a deficient superego is certainly not the same as an inhibited neurotic. Still, we may regard the inner conflicts of the psychopath and the neurotic in the same theoretical light. It seems to me that the juxtaposition introduced by Anna Freud (1959), that of defect and conflict, may be applied with much advantage to our difficult problem.

(c) When clinicians are asked why they describe a patient as psychopathic one can often discern in their answers that they perceive a "defect" in the patient. The defect can be constitutional, or caused by an organic illness, or by neglect in early infancy; in each case something is missing. Kraus (1947) pointed out that psychopathic manifestations may occur as residuals of a psychosis and are in that case based on a defect. Much can be absent from the neurotic personality's emotional life, as in the case of the compulsive-obsessive patient, who appears to be devoid of feelings. However, this inability to feel is based on a conflict and it is not a defect, or at most only a symptomatic defect. Some insist on interpreting all psychopathic defects as results of defense and conflict. I believe that is an error, and one should never lose sight of the fact that the psychogenic origin of a pathological deviation by no means implies its reversibility. Psychogenic factors lead not only to unconscious conflicts, but also to defects. This is the case particularly in very young persons. Regrettably the problem psychopathy-neuroses-psychoses arouses strong affective responses. Defective is for many identical with not treatable. But that is not correct; one must, however, use a technique different from that which resolves unconscious conflicts. Having attached an a priori idea of unsuitability for therapy to the concept of psychopathy, one is likely to reject the concept. Personal affective problems may also interfere with an unbiased evaluation of the concept. Defense mechanisms designed to disavow one's own psychopathic traits will lead one to miss the presence of a psychopathic defect in a patient, and to declare all of his behavior as neurotic. It also happens that psychiatrists think of a patient as a psychopath when they feel frightened by the patient's aggressive attitudes. They can thus avoid the question whether an error of their own may have been responsible for the patient's behavior; for instance, their having provoked the patient. In this way they escape criticism and at the same time gratify their own aggressive needs.

I should like to stress that acceptance or rejection of the concept of psychopathy does not depend on one's particular psychiatric school. It is possible that psychiatrists of Kraepelinian persuasion have a predilection for the constitutional origin of psychopathy. This constitutional bias has caused considerable confusion about the concept. There are, however, many analysts and dynamically and genetically oriented psychiatrists who also do not wish to dispense with the category of psychopathy.

In practice it will be necessary to determine the degree and the intensity of conflict and defect. In some cases only a psychoanalytic investigation can ascertain whether we deal with a defect or the consequences of a conflict. Neurotic conflicts sometimes take place on the matrix of a defect, and defects can prevent the healthy solution of a conflict.

Is there a correlation between the alloplastic reaction and personality defects caused by constitutional factors, organic illness or neglect in early childhood? Much can be adduced to support the assumption of such a correlation. Defects have a disturbing influence on the instinctual life and become manifest in damage to the ego functions; the ego's regulatory and integrative functions are impaired, the real world cannot be distinguished from the world of fantasy, and impulsive behavior is a common result. The definitions given under the headings (b) and (c) are often combined into one and this combination provides a suitable and meaningful concept of psychopathy. We speak of psychopathy when a patient displays disturbed alloplastic reactions, which often are of an asocial or dissocial nature; or when he inflicts pain on others on the basis of a personality defect, which has its roots in developmental disturbances. These are based on psychogenic and/or organic and constitutional factors. Thus we have reached a fruitful point of departure for further investigation, the direction of which is indicated by our adherence to the principle of multiple causations. The question as to the extent of the relative contributive factors arises. The answer to this question provides us with the guidelines for our therapeutic intervention. The general aim of the therapeutic effort is to improve the physical, particularly the cerebral functions, to strengthen the ego, and, if possible, to resolve unconscious conflicts. Before we discuss further the dynamics and genesis of psychopathy, let us attempt the delineation of the neurotic and psychopathic disorders from the psychoses.

While the neuroses and psychopathy represent forms of adaptation difficulties on the basis of developmental disturbances, instinctual conflicts and defects (in psychopathy), the psychoses can be described as forms of disadaptation. This concept has been used by Selye, Menninger, Prick, and Calon. The disadaptation affects primarily the ego functions: The manifestations of psychoses are primarily determined by disturbances of perception and of consciousness; not infrequently these are the result of an illness of the organic substratum. The unity of the personality is lost, the adaptation to the world is not only rendered diffcult, but impossible. The patient can no longer function in his familiar environment. The reality testing function fails, the distinction of the real world from the world governed by fantasy, wish and anxiety is no longer possible. The patient hallucinates; delusions supplant perceptions of the real world. Many neurotic and psychopathic persons also misperceive reality. They have their "private delusion," to use Lampl-de Groot's expression. The delusional images of the psychotic are, however, more intensely conscious, they invade the patient's conscious experience, are not kept concealed and indicate an extensive loss of contact with reality. The criteria for psychoses are disturbances of consciousness and of perception, hallucinations, and a diffuse borderline between the real and fantasied world.

Finally a few remarks about the differentiation between neuroses, psychopathy and the perversions.

We speak of perversion when the predominant symptom consists of abnormal sexual behavior, which prevents the normal instinctual gratification. The distinction introduced by Freud (1905) makes it possible to bring order into the realm of the perversions. He distinguished disturbances in respect to the instinctual object, and in respect to the instinctual aim. He writes in the first of the *Three Essays on the Theory of Sexuality:* "Let us call the person from whom sexual attraction proceeds the *sexual object* and the act towards which the instinct tends *the sexual aim*" (pp. 135–136). Deviations in respect to the sexual object for the adult are persons of the same sex (homosexuality), children, corpses (necrophilia), animals (sodomy) and articles of clothing or parts of the body (fetishism). We speak of deviation in respect to the sexual aim when sexual gratification is not sought and found with a partner of the other sex through union of the genital organs, but instead other organs take the place of the genitals as, for instance, the mouth or anus. Freud (1905) spoke of perversions as "sexual activities which . . . extend, in an anatomical sense, beyond the regions of the body that are designed for sexual union . . ." (p. 150). We also speak of perversion when component drives, i.e., instinctual impulses instead of being preliminary or auxiliary participants in the sexual union wholly dominate the person's sexual experience. When the main gratification is provided by rendering the partner helpless, or by inflicting pain we refer to that gratification as sadism. The passive counterpart to sadism is masochism. Exhibitionism is manifested by a compulsion to display one's genitalia, and voyeurism by the overwhelming desire to look at parts of the body which have some sexual significance or at sexual activities performed by others. We repeat: Perversion exists only when component instincts directed at anatomical extensions interfere with the achievement of orgasm normally, or when an object other than the normal stimulates the sexual drive.

Freud established the connection between infantile sexuality and perversions. He thought initially that the neurotic person wards off all aspects of the perverse experience. For instance blushing wards off exhibitionistic impulses, street phobia represents defense against masochistically tinged fantasies of prostitution. "Neuroses are . . . the negative of perversions" (p. 165) was Freud's formulation. Since then we have learned that perversion also has a defensive function. The male homosexual patient wards off hostility towards the man or neurotic anxieties related to the woman. Anal and oral gratifications are being sought to avoid castration anxiety. Other than the normal objects are sought because the normal object is proscribed by taboos. Component drives gain the upper hand in order to escape the neurotically dreaded adult sexual relationship. Viewed in this light perversion and neuroses are related. Pathological manifestations in both instances are the outcome of defense activity. Perversions and psychopathy are related in the sense that in both the patients tend to act out their instinctual impulses. Clinically we can divide perversions into two groups: (1) Those which in many ways resemble neuroses. The patients have a severe superego, an ego ideal with lofty expectations, relatively adequate ego functions, and a moderate tendency to act out. The perversion is mostly limited to fantasies, and only seldom acted out. In that case the action is followed by intense feelings of guilt. Social adaptation is adequate. In these cases the perversion is structured in analogy to a neurotic symptom. Many patients in this group effectively conceal their pathology. The accompanying character features of these people are mostly neurotic in nature; exhibitionists often are shy and inhibited. (2) The second group is related to psychopathy. They have a strong tendency to act out. They have had a distorted ego development and there are defects in the structure of their superego and ego ideal. One can call the members of this group impulse-driven psychopaths. Either gratification of the drive or defense against it can predominate in a given perversion. It is particularly the defense function of the perversion which makes understandable its compelling character. Experienced clinicians like Silleris-Smitt have stated that perverse impulses are always stronger than the normal.

We shall discuss the neuroses much more comprehensively than the perversions. Thorough acquaintance with the dynamics and genetics of neuroses and psychopathy will prove helpful in understanding one's perverse patients. Perversion represents flight, flight to other objects or to former forms of libidinal gratification—a regression. The use of the term object in this connection does not mean that the emotional life of people with perversions is entirely devoid of what has been called the "higher feelings." Fixations and regressions of the aggressive drive not connected with sexual activity are not perversions. The addicts, like the perverse, sometimes display similarities with neurotic or psychopathic persons. We shall discuss the psychology of addiction in a subsequent chapter.

DELINEATION AND CLASSIFICATION
OF NEUROTIC DISORDERS

We have differentiated the neurotic disturbances from the psychopathies and the psychoses. We must now undertake a classification of the neuroses. We cannot offer a classification as elegant as the periodic table of the elements, or as neatly arranged as the classifications of descriptive biology, but we can provide a serviceable classification by approaching the clinical and descriptive material from the dynamic and genetic points of view.

It is natural that we find in psychoanalytic literature a classification which is oriented along the lines of libidinal development. I shall quite intentionally make use of both the psychiatric and the psychoanalytic points of view. Ever since psychoanalysis has systematically investigated ego, superego and ego ideal and their connections with the drives, this approach in my opinion has proven the most productive of all. We must point out an element of danger here. Since in psychoanalytic usage many concepts have had their original meaning changed, one must agree beforehand on the meaning one wishes a given concept to have. For example, the concept of hysteria is burdened with considerable confusion. The manifestations of hysteria have been known for a long time. Freud discovered that hysteria is based on regression of fixation to the phallic phase of libidinal development, owing to a failure of the resolution of the Oedipus complex. Later it was ascertained that many disease manifestations and character deformations have an internal structure not unlike that of hysteria. Neurotic entities related to hysteria were thus delineated, such as the characters described by Abraham (1920), whose difficulties were rooted in their inability to accept their existence as women.

Many psychoanalysts and psychiatrists call all these entities hysteria, even though at first glance they do not at all resemble the familiar picture of hysteria. If consideration is given to the unconscious processes, one will tend to name all those neuroses hysterical which issue from the phallic problems and manifest themselves in sexual difficulties. This application of our knowledge of unconscious processes to the diagnosis is not easily comprehensible for the young psychiatrist in training. Those who favor descriptive and phenomenological differentiations will not welcome this broadening of the concepts of hysteria. In my opinion it is advisable to reserve the diagnosis of hysteria for the condition manifested by conversion symptoms, anxiety, disturbances of consciousness and the character traits of infantilism, artificiality, egocentricity and self-importance. The other neurotic conditions related to hysteria we shall call hysterical neuroses or neuroses with hysterical features. Whatever the words we employ, confusion can only be avoided if we make clear from the beginning what meaning we intend to ascribe to them.

We must familiarize ourselves with the manifestations of neurotic illness, and also with the explanation of their nature provided by the study of the relevant unconscious processes. Most psychiatrists prefer one or the other approach, but, here as in other fields, making the best of two worlds promises the most enlightenment. As in hysteria, the Oedipus complex is the nuclear problem even in those neuroses in which one is impressed with the regression to the pregenital phases of the development of the libido. One can observe with increasing clarity that especially in cases in which the pregenital phase had an uneven course the Oedipus complex forms an impassable barrier to further development. Developmental disturbances, fixations and regressions to the different phases can be demonstrated in these cases. There are neuroses in which the phallic, anal or oral traits completely dominate the picture and the genesis of the neuroses. We shall clarify all this in the course of our study.

Neurotic manifestations must be evaluated not only in terms of the fixations and regressions in the realm of the instinctual strivings, but also in terms of the disturbances of the ego functions, and the defense mechanisms. A diagnosis of hysteria, compulsive neurosis, etc., will not satisfy the person who wants to gain real insight into the neuroses or perversions. He will attempt to estimate the seriousness and the degree of the disturbance. In one case the deviations may be limited in scope, in another they may destroy the person's life. To arrive at an indication for therapy and a prognosis one has to estimate the patient's potentialities, his gifts, abilities, skills, and intellectual capacities. What has he accomplished in life, is he able to work, does he have a meaningful hobby, does he have personal relationships which give him some partial, if not optimal, gratification? We are interested in the intensity and the scope of his disturbances. This brings us again to the ego functions.

A large number of neurotics and perverts have a more or less adequate adaptation though some of their ego functions are impaired by the neurotic conflict. The instinctual conflicts cause a misreading of reality. The hysteric misconstrues reality because of his defense through repression. The compulsive does it through his adherence to magical thinking. Some patients maintain only limited contact with reality. When their inner tensions rise they are in danger of chaotic reaction. Lampl-de Groot believes that in these cases the ego has remained in an early stage of development. There is not only a regression or fixation to infantile instinctual gratification, but also an arrested ego development. As a result, reality testing, tolerance of frustration and the ego's capacity of integration fail under internal or external stress. At this point we are reminded of the distinction between defect and conflict. It is not surprising that we think of psychopathy or psychosis in cases with a weak or distorted ego. But these psychotic manifestations quickly disappear, as does the psychopathic behavior, and we have again a patient whom we correctly diagnose as neurotic. Patients like these are often called borderline cases. We are not content with making the diagnosis of hysteria, perversion etc. In addition our aim is to establish how the person's ego performs, which areas of his life are relatively free from pathology, and if his conflicts invariably result in failures, or also in some successes. Some neurotic persons are unable to study and learn, others study excessively. It is of great importance to establish whether a person is capable of extending effort and asserting himself, or whether his inner tensions render him helpless and result in his failure. Gifted persons are more prone to sublimate internal tensions than the less gifted. Character and neuroses must be viewed in their mutual relationship. Naturally the neurosis has a significant effect on what a person does with his gifts, but his gifts also play a significant role in what the person does with his neurosis. In that connection, attention is called to Dr. Frijung-Schreuder's (1964/65) essay on Balzac.

The attitude of the patient to his illness is of great importance for the indications for our therapeutic intervention. Even though we put much emphasis on the degree of severity of the neurosis, a classification in which we combine clinical, descriptive, dynamic and genetic points of view is indispensable. We shall deal with the classical syndrome of hysteria, with the neuroses related to hysteria in the woman, the so-called inhibited type, and the characters described by Abraham, which are conditioned by a neurotic response to the anatomical difference in the sexes. The classical hysterical character and the inhibited type occur in men as well as in women. We shall further consider the neurotic symptoms and character formations connected with the passive-feminine attitude: The so-called phallic-narcisstic type, the "Don Juan" type, also the "Don Juan of success," and the character formations which are conspicuous by their difficulties with authorities and by work disturbances. Passive homosexuality will be mentioned in this connection though it properly belongs among the perversions. The masochistic character disturbances are related to these forms of neuroses.

We shall then proceed to a study of the anxiety neuroses, the phobias, the neuroses with derealization and depersonalization. Within the context of the compulsive-obsessive neuroses we shall also examine the psychasthenic personality.

The dynamic and genetic points of view not only enable us to understand the neurotic symptoms, they also afford us insight into the neurotic character formations. Many character types were not even recognized and described until we studied them in this new light. The same is true of the recognition of the function of character as defense. These character types can be arranged in a system oriented along the phases of libidinal development. In the course of studying them it became evident that the different phases are participating in characteristic ways in the development of specific character deformations.

In our classification of the neuroses we shall also use the description of character entities arrived at by other than psychoanalytic ways of thinking. We adopt these descriptions because they are of importance in our daily practice. Is this an expression of clinical eclecticism? Not at all. It is an attempt to proceed systematically in practice as well as in theory. We shall attempt to give a dynamic and genetic interpretation of important character formations known to clinical psychiatry, among them those of the neurasthenic and of the sensitive character. Finally, let us repeat: The investigation of clinical manifestations must be associated with insight into the unconscious processes. We remind ourselves of a word by Kant: Description without consideration of dynamic and genetic processes is blind. A theory of the neuroses which neglects to examine man in the multiplicity of the constituent aspects of his personality and sees only isolated mechanisms cannot be a useful tool.

3

HYSTERIA AND RELATED NEUROSES

Hysteria is undoubtedly the best known among the neuroses. The term has fallen into ill-repute because it has been used pejoratively. In Dutch vernacular the word is also used to indicate hypersexuality. For others hysterical is identical with pretense or malingering. In scientific usage the word hysteria has none of these meanings.

Originally the term hysteria was used for an illness in which the main symptoms were conversion and disturbances of consciousness. Freud discovered that fixation and regression to the phallic phase initiated by an unresolved Oedipus complex represented an important causal factor in the genesis of hysteria. In time all those neuroses were called hysterical which had in common with hysteria unresolved oedipal problems and fixation and/or regression to the phallic stage. Many combinations of symptoms and character deformations which had little resemblance to the psychiatric disease entity of hysteria were then also called hysterical. The naming of a disease rests so often on custom or usage. In my view, it does not appear desirable to broaden the concept of hysteria to such an extent. The following classification seems clinically serviceable and theoretically justified.

We find the following symptoms in the classical syndrome

of hysteria: Conversions and disturbances of consciousness, as its nuclear symptoms; a variety of nonspecific symptoms associated with these such as anxiety, sexual dysfunctions like frigidity and impotence, inferiority feelings and others.

We speak of a hysterical character when the following qualities are present: Histrionic behavior, affectation, infantilism and egocentricity. Often the need to get attention is added to this list. A characteristic feature of hysterics is the wish to experience and express more than they are capable of; they exaggerate everything in an attempt to appeal to others. Klages called attention to this tension differential between inner helplessness and exaggerated need for expression.

This trait of hysterical patients manifests itself in their use of language. They enjoy using as many superlatives as possible. Words like terrible, horrible, indescribable, unspeakable and fantastic are overused.

In connection with the discussion of hysteria we shall add some dynamically and genetically oriented observations on some common neurotic manifestations of a general character, such as feelings of exhaustion, lability and inadequacy. One not infrequently encounters these reactions associated with hysteria.

CONVERSION SYMPTOMS

Our first subjects are the occasionally spectacular manifestations of conversion which tend to irritate the physician who is saturated with materialistic prejudices acquired in his training. His patients complain bitterly, yet "there is nothing wrong with them." What is meant by this phrase? In every instance this is a formulation connected with the erroneous once-held view that all illness is somatic. The contemporary concept of illness is that it is a disturbance of adaptation. A conversion symptom is no less tormenting than the symptom of an organic illness, and hysteria, the disease at the root of the conversion is often more serious and more difficult to treat than many organic diseases.

What is a conversion symptom? It is the expression of a psychic conflict in the form of a disturbance of a bodily function, in pain or in other unpleasant sensations. The number of patients with conversion symptoms a doctor may see depends on the kind of practice he maintains. Intellectual patients usually have other complaints than conversion symptoms, though their neuroses may be hysterical or related to hysteria. It is apparently easier for a person of simple mentality to produce conversion symptoms. However, conversion symptoms are never entirely lacking even in the cases of sophisticated persons whose only complaint is a chronic discontent and unhappiness in life.

It is advisable to differentiate the concept of conversion from functional, hypochondrical and psychosomatic complaints. "Functional" is the wider concept; many conversion symptoms are functional in nature, but not every functional disturbance is a conversion symptom. Functional means a disturbed function not caused by pathological organic processes. For instance, functional headaches need not be a conversion symptom, however, a headache can express the idea that one's head is bursting. Similarly, hysterical vomiting may be a communication as the following: "I am sick of it, I cannot bear it, I am too full of it."

Conversion must also be differentiated from hypochondria. The hypochondriacal attitude is one of conscious preoccupation with the body, a morbid concern with it, which can find expression in different psychic areas (Ladee, 1961). The hypochondriacal patient has strange sensations, he believes he suffers from a disease and worries about it. One could of course raise the question whether hypochondriacal ruminations are part of every conversion symptom. We find however that many hysterical patients have a rather indifferent attitude to their conversion symptoms, at least as far as their conscious experience is concerned. We speak of the *"belle indifférence"* of hysterical patients. Sometimes the conversion symptom appears more or less split off from the rest of the personality, but there certainly are conversion symptoms which are accompanied by hypochondriacal feelings. When hypochondriacal elements dominate the picture the conversion symptom loses much of its significance for the diagnosis, and we look for clarification in other directions. In addition conversion must be differentiated from the organ-neurotic symptoms which lack the feature of expressing an idea which is present in conversion symptoms. The organ-neurotic symptoms are manifestations accompanying psychic tension, for instance, anxiety. A rapid pulse rate and vague but disturbing sensations in the region of the heart are equivalents of anxiety. In many cases the differentiation can be in dispute.

It is certainly advisable to pay attention to the differences between conversion and psychosomatic symptoms. In the latter, the psychic tensions have resulted in objectively discernible results of disturbed functions, i.e., in morphological changes. A well-known example is the peptic ulcer. Certain symptoms can simultaneously have the character of a conversion symptom and of a psychosomatic phenomenon. This fact does not vitiate their differentiation.

We can dispense with a listing of all possible conversion symptoms. They are always a compromise formation between a derivative of the drive and the defense directed against it. Their significance, like that of symbols in the dream, is undoubtedly dependent upon the context in which they appear. There is no dictionary of language of the organs.

Stomach aches often express the complaint: "I cannot cope with what is happening to me." Abdominal pain is often related to sexual disturbances, and backaches to the feeling: "The burden of life is too heavy for me." The well-known hysterical paralyses most often represent punishment and the wish to be helped. Hysterical dizziness can express the fear of falling, in the symbolic sense of a "fallen woman." Hysterical blindness is a well-known conversion symptom, and so are many symptoms affecting the sympathetic nervous system, e.g., nausea, vomiting, and cardiac palpitation with or without the accompanying fear of death. The well-known astasia and abasia of the hysterical patient often express the thoughts: "I cannot stand on my own feet, I cannot move through life on my own." A foul or bitter taste in the mouth reveals its meaning easily.

Discussions of conversion symptoms always include the possibility that patients with hysterical cardiac complaints may have coronary disease, or those with hysterical abdominal pain may suffer from appendicitis, and that these conditions, if neglected, may have a fatal outcome. No one doubts these facts: they are a good reason for caution and a reminder not to make the diagnosis of conversion too hastily—certainly not on the basis of the negative findings of a physical examination alone. The diagnosis of conversion in a hysterical neurosis must be based on positive criteria. Hysteria is a psychiatric diagnosis which should never be made solely on the basis of the absence of somatic deviations from the norm.

All too often conversion symptoms are ascribed to pretense and malingering. Malingering or feigning illness is an intentional deceptive activity, while a conversion symptom is an unconsciously motivated genuine disturbance of function. It is more appropriate to compare the conversion symptom to amblyopia, a symptom familiar to the ophthalmologist. Amblyopia is a lack of perception in spite of a sound visual apparatus. The patient with strabismus suppresses the disturbing image. The analogy with repression is remarkably close because in both instances the suppression occurs as a result of a conflict. One speaks of a conflict between the two retinal images. In ambloyopia we have a genuine defect of a function; the person does not see in spite of the presence of an anatomically sound organ.[1] The conversion symptoms must be viewed in the same light, and not as pretense.

DISTURBANCES OF CONSCIOUSNESS

The most conspicuous though not the most important of the disturbances of consciousness is the hysterical attack. The disturbances of self-awareness, as for instance depersonalization and the derealization associated with it, occur more commonly and last longer than hysterical attacks. The hysterical attack can resemble an epileptic seizure (I must defer to the textbooks of neurology for the differential diagnosis). It can be stated that a hysterical attack always represents either a conflict or a wish-fulfillment. A limited contact with the surrounding world, i.e., with a person or persons of significance for the patient, continues throughout the attack. The amnesia covering the event can often be lifted. The hysterical twilight state can present a problem in differential diagnosis in regard to the state of impaired consciousness of the epileptic. The observation that epileptic twilight states can be caused by affective forces further increases the difficulties of the differentiation. Epileptic twilight states show a conspicuous similarity to hysterical twilight states—a circumstance open to interesting speculations. We must re-emphasize, however, that the possibility of organic disorders has to be kept in mind whenever twilight states or other disturbances of consciousness enter the clinical picture. One often hears elaborate tales about large cerebral tumors found in allegedly hysterical patients. Most of these reports are spurious. Nevertheless it is imperative to examine the patient thoroughly.

Many hysterical patients give the impression that they are subject to frequent disturbances of consciousness. Nurses ob-

[1] I am grateful to Professor A. Hagedorn for suggesting this analogy.

serving the patient may report that "they don't seem to be all there." One notes that this dull "absence" quickly disappears when some strong emotional appeal is made to the patient. The patient is submerged in only vaguely conscious day-dreams, or in unconscious fantasies and this gives him the air of numbness. In general it can be stated that hysterical patients tolerate poorly the present, the here and now of life. They live in the past or in the future.

SEXUAL DISTURBANCES

One of the symptoms indicative of sexual conflict is impotence, or frigidity. Disturbances of sexual function can be listed among the conversion symptoms, but sexual disturbances are to be found outside of the framework of classical hysteria as well. Sexual disturbances are common aspects of many neuroses. Vaginism, a spasm of the adductor muscles and of the muscles of the female genital organ clearly expresses that the patient does not wish to have sexual intercourse with a man. Often impotence and frigidity give the impression of deficiency. We can say that the prohibitions of the superego produce a deficient function. These symptoms occur very frequently. Frigidity is almost always one of the symptoms of clinical hysteria. Of course, there are also cases of hysteria without impairment of the capacity to experience an orgasm, but the sexual function is not completely integrated into the personality. Many authorities, following W. Reich, consider sexual potency and capacity to experience orgasm as the most important criterion of mental health. Impotence is indeed an essential neurotic symptom; yet undisturbed sexual potency is no proof of health. Severe neuroses can run their course without impairing either potency or orgastic capacity. Hartmann[2] concurs with me in this view. The separation into sensuality on one side, and tender-

[2] Personal communication.

ness and companionship on the other is not restricted to men. In many women capacity for orgasm and ability to love by no means coincide. In the clinical picture of classical hysteria frigidity is always a symptom of "phallic hysteria."

In disturbances of the male sexual potency we distinguish the failure to have an erection from the failure to ejaculate the seminal fluid. Premature ejaculation can occur either before or very shortly after entry of the penis into the vagina.

It is of fundamental significance for the diagnostic classification of the neuroses as well as for the general knowledge of man to view sexuality and its disturbances not as isolated entities, but in conjunction with a full consideration of the person and his or her social and personal relationships. The neurotic person may be capable of an orgasm, yet incapble of love. At least, not in the full sense of the word. The word love is misleading. Aldous Huxley has pointed out that one can say "I love this flower," and also "I love ice cream." Love of the flower implies that we admire its unfolding and wish it to endure. We consume the ice cream. The statement that one loves often means only that one expects sexual gratification. The personality of the partner and his essential interests are then of little concern, a clear case of "ice-cream love." To feel sheltered in someone's presence, to find gratification of sexual needs, may, but need not be aspects of love in the full sense of that word. These wishes and needs may even be destructive for the partner insofar as he or she is used or misused solely as the supplier of instinctual gratification.

Disturbances of the ability to love demonstrate most clearly that unresolved problems stemming from all stages of development are responsible for the disorder. Inhibitions and repression, false modesty, the incapacity to give, excessive dependency, which the Anglo-Saxons so appropriately term "dependent and demanding," can all interfere with the forming of mature love relationships. The sexual disorders proper are also influenced by factors connected with the different phases of libidinal development.

Frigidity can be the result of unconscious guilt feelings because of unresolved problems of adolescent masturbation. It then is an inhibition intended to ward off the forbidden incestuous oedipal feelings for the father. Frigidity can also have the meaning of refusal to experience pleasure at the sites of excretion, based on conflicts rooted in the anal phase. Finally, as a derivative of the early oral phase, it can express the refusal to sustain the partner with one's love and to give him a feeling of security and comfort. Bergler (1946) believes that the oral conflicts are the main cause of impotence. That may be true in some cases, however, it is a mistake to hold one single factor responsible for the total problem. We see in this example how some investigators are inclined to isolate one element of psychoanalytic theory and disregard all others. One is exclusively preoccupied with the preoedipal period; the other sees only inferiority feelings, etc. Such a way of looking at a problem is always too one-sided and fails to recognize the complexity of the problems with which life confronts us.

What was said here in regard to frigidity applies to every neurotic symptom in which problems from different stages of development find expression. A work inhibition can be caused by the fear of ridicule because praise and success are never experienced as sufficient; it can be related to exhibitionistic problems; it can be the result of an inability to listen to an order, obedience being thought of as weakness; it can be based on a stubborn opposition to orders stemming from the anal period, and finally on the inability to give love because of the wish to take revenge on the mother who has forced one to "go hungry" in childhood. Often it is necessary to trace and work through all these determinants of a symptom if one wishes to bring about its resolution.

The preceding remarks make clear that the investigation of

the sexual dysfunctions must not be isolated from the examination of the total personality. Sexual life involves the total person, without necessarily absorbing it. The evaluation of disturbances of a person's sexual power should extend to questions concerning his capability of experiencing feelings of companionship, tenderness and love in a lasting relationship. The study of neuroses leads here to sociocultural and anthropological subjects. Is it normal that we feel unhappy when a gratifying love relationship is absent from our life, or should professional activity or activity in other areas of life make up for the lack? Does contemporary man expect to find in his love relationship much of what was formerly found in religion, namely the experience of the meaningfullness of life and the ability to bear the thought of its limits and of death? Do we expect too much from sexual gratification, namely not alone gratification but general peace of mind? The answers to these questions rest more on our *Weltanschauung* and our wishes than on results of empirical investigation. It should never be forgotten that intense sexual needs may serve to ward off different impulses and feelings. The lack of sexual fulfillment can be neurotically motivated, but so can an exaggerated sexual activity. We regard as mentally healthy a person who functions in an integrated way, and in whose life everything has both an absolute and a relative significance.

ANXIETY

Anxiety is the expectation of an unknown evil, a menace that does not issue from something definite in the environment, but from the world in its undefined totality. Except in phobias, where anxiety is related to a specific situation, anxiety is diffuse, irrational and ill-suited to serve as an adaptive defense. As with the feeling of guilt we must distinguish between neurotic and "adaptive" anxiety. What is essential is how we deal with our anxiety. The differentiation between neurotic and healthy anxiety appears even more difficult than the distinction between neurotic and normal feelings of guilt. We must again caution against working with abstract standards of normality which are not patterned by empirical science, but by a very personal image of people shaped by the influence of our own anxieties, by our defenses against anxiety, and by our wishful thinking.

Science and our philosophy of life should mutually enrich each other, but we must not lose track of the limitations of each. It seems to me that many contemporary existential views about human beings raise a chronic neurotic anxiety to the status of normality (Huehnerfeld, 1959). Metaphysical significance is ascribed to a series of neurotic symptoms, to sexual inhibition, inhibition of aggression, anxiety, depersonalization, and warded-off emotions. Anxiety must be designated as neurotic when it has a disintegrating effect, when it weakens the internal synthesis, and causes us to avoid situations in which we are challenged to make the effort to mature.

There exists also a pathological absence of anxiety. Cleckley (1955) pointed out that certain psychopathic persons show remarkably little anxiety in situations in which the person whose thoughts and feelings are normal would experience anxiety. We see no reason to provide neurotic anxiety with a metaphysical halo, and it makes just as little sense to proclaim the incapacity to experience anxiety as the new ideal. Conscious or unconscious anxiety plays a significant role in the difficulties of all our patients. In some instances we observe the anxiety directly, in others we observe the symptoms and character deformations caused by the ego's efforts to ward off anxiety. We distinguish realistic anxiety, in situations of great external danger; superego anxiety, when we act or wish to act against the standards of our conscience; and id anxiety, the fear of instinctual impulses. It seems to me that the primary anxiety in which all later anxiety has its roots is the anxiety that overwhelms the infant when he is left to himself. We experience anxiety when warded off instinctual impulses seek to enter consciousness and press towards actions which were once forbidden by the parents and are still forbidden by their intrapsychic representative, the superego. It was originally felt by the child when he was threatened by the loss of his parents' love. In the genesis and the dynamics of all neurotic disorders anxiety plays a significant role. This is true whether the anxiety is consciously experienced or not. In some neurotic conditions anxiety is the most conspicuous symptom. When the anxiety is diffuse, we are dealing with an anxiety neurosis. The latter is characterized by pervasive inner tension and free-floating anxiety, i.e., a constant readiness to experience anxiety. Freud considered the anxiety neuroses as one of the "actual" neuroses, and ascribed an important causative role to coitus interruptus. I observed that indeed anxiety occurs in situations of sudden sexual abstinence. That is not, however, the only cause of anxiety; in addition, a neurotic disposition has to be present. We shall use the term anxiety neurosis for conditions in which pervasive anxiety is the most conspicuous neurotic symptom.

In most neuroses the consequences of anxiety are character deformations and the formation of extensive systems of defense. When the defense has been mitigated in the course of psychoanalytic treatment the original anxiety sometimes reappears on the surface. The process of the development of the neurosis then reverses itself. The neurosis becomes converted into an anxiety neurosis, and the last phase of the therapeutic psychoanalysis consists of treating this resurrected anxiety neurosis. Often the anxiety surges up together with memories of those traumatic situations which played a significant part in the genesis of the neurosis. One of my patients in whose neurosis castration fears were the dominant pathogenic factor, experienced before his final recovery a period of intense fear of the color red, i.e., the color of blood.

He objected to his wife's red dresses and her red lipstick. Another patient developed a typical anxiety neurosis just before he was able to recall the sexual feelings he once had felt towards his brother. During this period he had a strong need to be near someone who could understand his predicament. Once again we remind ourselves that anxiety can be an extremely painful symptom, often worse than physical pain, and that we must do everything in our power to relieve the patient of his anxiety. If anxiety arises in the course of "revelational" therapy, we must advise the patient to bear his anxiety, since its suppression is likely to retard the process of recovery. The patient who trusts his physician, and knows that his anxiety can be relieved will tolerate very intense anxiety. When one considers how tormenting, even unbearable, anxiety can be it is understandable that a fear of it can develop. Anxiety-ridden patients often display a beseeching and dependent attitude, a sign of their partial regression. They constantly want someone near them, ask someone to hold their hand, to sit near them, etc.

When anxiety is the presenting symptom of a hysterical neurosis we can speak of anxiety hysteria. Fenichel (1931) states: "In anxiety hysteria, however, the anxiety is specifically connected with a special situation, which represents the danger situation." Here he designates as anxiety hysteria a neurosis which other writers call phobia. The phobic fears are connected with very specific situations: fear of crossing the street, of open places, of heights, of examinations, of speaking in public, etc. One must not conclude that the label anxiety hysteria implies that the feeling of anxiety is not genuine.

Another group of phobias is that of the anticipatory anxieties. To this group belong erythrophobia, (fear of blushing), fear of fainting, fear of making a bad impression in society, etc. Furthermore we are acquainted with phobias associated with specific objects which have a symbolic character and are prone to stimulate instinctual impulses—blood, knives, dirt, small and large animals are such objects. The phobia of little Hans, his fear of a horse, was described by Freud (1909), and has become famous.

Hysterical patients often have an exaggerated fear of specific animals. Such phobias lie between anxiety and compulsion, i.e., compulsive avoidance can have the purpose of warding off anxiety. It is therefore not astonishing to find phobias in the neuroses which have something in common with both hysteria and obsessive-compulsive neurosis.

When anxiety reaches a certain degree of intensity, it is often accompanied by somatic reactions, such as sweating, tachycardia, trembling, or diarrhea. These symptoms in turn increase the anxiety. Anxiety can also evoke a hypochondriacal response. Cardiac neuroses are often caused by intense feelings of guilt, the patients fear that the sentence of death will be meted out to them.

In summary, I want to emphasize the significance of anxiety for neurotic symptom formation, for the genesis of character deformations, neurotic maneuvers and neurotic relationships. All of these are in the service of warding off anxiety which originates in infantile and childhood experiences.

FEELINGS OF GUILT AND INFERIORITY

Feelings of guilt and inferiority play a large role in hysterical neuroses: this, of course, does not imply their absence in other neuroses. We shall review these phenomena in detail. Freud made the discovery that hysteria is a consequence of unresolved oedipal problems. Hence, the presence of conscious and unconscious guilt feelings is not surprising. In many cases, the feeling of guilt results in an intense need for punishment. To avoid the experience of painful anxiety, one must atone for the forbidden fantasies. Neurotic guilt leads to a continuation of the ill-adapted behavior and to a further disruption of the synthetic and integrative functions of the ego. For example, a young man is tormented by guilt feelings because of masturbation. The guilt feelings cause a chronic depressive mood, and, in order to escape this mood, he is driven to seek gratification in more masturbation. His sexuality cannot be integrated into his personality structure. His interpersonal relationships are disturbed by his fear of punishment and attitude of distrust. In contrast, normal guilt motivates us to repair the damage inflicted and to avoid the repetition of undesirable actions. To illustrate: a healthy young woman who has had a sexual affair with a man whom she does not love feels guilty but is able to bring the affair to an end, and looks forward to a relationship in which sexuality, tenderness and companionship will be fully integrated.

The severe and inappropriately functioning superego condemns the neurotic and his exalted ego ideal creates feelings of inferiority in him. The perception of his own inexpedient behavior and failure further increases the neurotic feeling of inferiority, and the perception of personal insufficiency aggravates the difficulties still more. I once heard someone say about a patient, "He does not feel inferior, he *is* inferior." This harsh and pitiless judgement was not entirely wrong. The neurosis does indeed prevent the person from realizing his potential. To feel insufficient is not a sign of modesty, but rather its neurotic opposite. Closer examination always reveals the presence of unconscious and vaguely conscious fantasies of grandeur. Self-adulation comes before self-depreciation. According to Nietzsche, "When man holds himself in contempt, he admires himself for so doing."

The problem of the neurotic feelings of guilt and insufficiency leads us to the narcissistic problems of the hysterical patient (Van der Waals, 1940). Narcissism means love of one's own person. We have to devote some discussion to this subject. Our self-esteem has several sources. We derive it from our good relationships with others, from the love which others feel for us, from our successes in work, from sexual gratification, from the fact that we command an adapted aggressivity, and particularly from an optimal relationship with our superego and ego ideal. This inner harmony, this peace of mind renders us independent of praise and scorn and enables us to assert ourselves in the world in a suitable manner. I should like to stress the importance of that inner harmony, not because of moralistic or philosophical considerations, but on the basis of empirical facts. Excessive dependence on the environment, anxious search for security, compulsive demand for sexual gratification, and the chase after success have their roots in the fact that the different areas of the personality are not well-integrated, and that we do not live in peace with ourselves.

The sources of self-esteem of hysterical patients are depleted and unproductive. Their interpersonal relationships are disturbed by feelings of insufficiency and inferiority and by projection of guilt and mistrust. They are further jeopardized by being permeated with repressed sexuality; there are no true sexual gratifications, and a constant superego conflict is present. The development of the aggressive drive has progressed no further than to quarrelsomeness and other irksome traits. All this presents the development of normal self-love and self-esteem. The patient is compelled to bolster his self-esteem in different ways. He relies on his fantasies, his false concept of self, and he misuses interpersonal relationships for narcissistic purposes. The last formulation requires some elaboration. We have already pointed out that interpersonal relationships gratify our narcissistic needs, i.e., increase our self-esteem. During early childhood the ego derives all its self-confidence from the love of the child's parents. After the formation of the superego the self-esteem becomes more independent of the parents and other people; in the superego the parents have become part of the personality. This process of internalization does not fully take place in neurotic persons, and consequently they remain dependent on others for the support of their self-esteem. Some neurotic patients use interpersonal relationships mainly for the build-up of their self-esteem. Men may manifest this in an abnormal need to be admired for accomplishments, in restless chasing after success, in the need to be spectacular at all costs. That these people are not concerned with the relationship in itself is clearly evident in their dropping friends as soon as they have experienced a mild frustration or as soon as someone else promises them richer rewards. Carp (1947) has described this pattern very well for the case of the hysterical seducer. These people, so friendly and cordial when they are out to conquer, are disappointing by virtue of the inconsiderate way in which they sacrifice the interests of others to their own interests. Yet they profess high ethical and moral beliefs. They create bitter enemies, and provoke even the therapist to forget occasionally that their behavior is the expression of a hysterical neurosis and that their emotional life is profoundly distorted. In women, narcissistic disturbances present themselves differently. While men look mainly to their profession for opportunities of narcissistic gratification, women seek narcissistic gratification in love relationships. There they seek replenishment and satisfaction of their narcissistic needs. Now we have proceeded from the discussion of neurotic symptoms to that of the neurotic character, neurotic relationships and maneuvers.

Need for punishment and feelings of guilt, particularly when they are unconscious, greatly influence interpersonal relationships. We can consider the manner in which a neurotic person, oppressed by his feelings of guilt, behaves in his relations with others. If one is constantly subjected to the accusations of the superego and cannot fulfill the demands of the ego ideal, one is particularly eager to be pronounced free of guilt by others; one wants to be loved by them and receive their praise as a counterweight against self-condemnation.

This is particularly true of the "sensitive character" type, to be discussed now.

The vulnerability of the sensitive may in part be constitutionally determined: Their hypersensitivity is such that even the slightest sign of disapproval is taken by them as proof of their worthlessness. The rejection, whether real or fantasied, is experienced as painful frustration, anger results, and because of the inhibition of their aggression this anger can neither be experienced nor acted upon; the unfortunate neurotic feels guiltier than ever, and demands with increasing intensity that his environment acquit him and absolve him of his guilt. The frustration tolerance is further weakened when the interpersonal relationships are also called upon to satisfy passive libidinal needs, the longing for care, security and affection. These mechanisms, though particularly conspicuous in sensitive personalities, are present in all hysterical neuroses. Excessive guilt feeling makes us excessively dependent on proof of love and esteem from the environment. There are, of course, other reactions to excessive unconscious guilt. Some people try to evoke the punishment which they believe they deserve; in such instances we refer to moral masochism.

The difference between neurotic symptoms and neurotic character is only relative. The feeling of inferiority can be viewed either as a symptom or a character anomaly. The decisive criterion is the degree to which the phenomenon is or is not ego-alien. Some patients with a hysterical neurosis consciously experience the painful aspects of their feelings of guilt and inferiority; others are entirely unaware of these feelings on the conscious level, and disclose their consequences only in the neurotic symptomatology.

DEREALIZATION AND DEPERSONALIZATION

What has been said about neurotic guilt and inferiority feelings also applies to the phenomenon of depersonalization. Of more signficance for the psychiatrist's daily practice than the obvious disturbances of consciousness are those subtle but worrisome lapses of awareness of the self and of reality, which do not come to the investigator's attention unless the patients tell him about them. These patients suffer from symptoms of derealization or depersonalization. A number of investigators maintain that every neurotic patient is to some degree subject to depersonalization. The patients complain of an inner emptiness, a sensation of not being able to feel anything. Whatever happens passes them by. One must not underestimate the suffering experienced by these patients. The psychiatrist who is familiar with the dynamics of the hysterical processes will not be surprised by the observation that the patients complain of not being able to experience the very feeling they would like to experience most, and cannot derive pleasure from what they are most eager to enjoy. Success at an examination fails to enhance the patient's pride; he feels like a disinterested spectator at a celebration; he experiences not joy, but the painful inability to experience joy. If not for that distressing sensation he would not even know that there is reason for contentment. A neurotic woman who spent years waiting, finally finds herself in her lover's arms. In despair she thinks, "I feel nothing!" She perceives the sexual climax like the performance of a mechanical contrivance. Such phenomena lose the aspect of mystery when we consider depersonalization and derealization as the internal perception of the result of repression. The appropriate affects have been removed from consciousness and the lack of this "existential" aspect of the experience is painful. We recognize from this description that depersonalization and derealization can be considered as disturbances of affect. They are not confined to hysterical neuroses. The frame of reference in which they are to be considered is a matter of diagnosis. When these disturbances are the central issue it is justified to speak of a depersonalization or derealization syndrome. The differential diagnosis is not easy; these symptoms can occur in the course of beginning schizophrenias and various exogenic and endogenic conditions, such as the postpartum psychoses and depressions.

The disturbances of consciousness are in many cases the result of a powerful defense against aggressive impulses. It should be pointed out in general that pathologic sexuality is not the sole cause of hysterical neuroses; the conflicts centered around aggression are no less important.

THE HYSTERICAL CHARACTER

The manifestations of the hysterical character most commonly mentioned are: exaggerated self-importance, egocentricity, infantilism, and a general artfulness. Several objections can be raised to this enumeration. The most important one is that these character traits are often not in the foreground of the total image of the person. Often the patients with a clearly hysterical symptomatology appear inhibited and retiring. We are familiar with the image of the quiet and shy girl, so desirable and exciting to many men, because her air of mystery, and her sphinxlike character lend themselves well to serve as a screen on which many diverse fantasies may be projected. The very essence of what the man so passionately desires appears hidden in her nature. The inhibited patient corresponds precisely to the somewhat obsolete ideal of the charming mysterious woman. Sociological and cultural factors were certainly influential in the formation of this image; it was expected that women quietly and modestly went about their tasks. Concealed behind this inhibition not infrequently are passionate sexual and aggressive fantasies. The three aspects of the hysterical character— egocentricity, infantile attitudes, and spuriousness—are also to be found in these patients.

I am not entirely convinced that the triad of features referred to above is correct, at least not in this rigid formulation. Egocentricity has a slightly moralizing aspect, infantilism says very little, and the lack of genuineness is associated with the false theory of a constitutional origin.

I shall begin with a few remarks about the infantile attitude. Every neurotic individual is infantile in a certain sense—the rigid compulsive neurotic, or the alcoholic, no less than the hysteric. The infantile behavior of the hysterical patient is composed of different elements. Descriptively we can say that the hysterical patient displays behavior patterns which we consider normal in the child, but ill-adapted in the adult, such as frequent pouting, quarrelsomeness, proneness to feel discriminated against, intense affective responses to trivial frustrations, and generally exaggerated reactions. It is by no means unusual for a hysterical patient to withdraw into his bedroom and feel injured and offended by a trivial incident which an average person would have ignored or resolved without difficulty. One often hears the opinion that this childish behavior has the sole purpose of bending the environment to the hysteric's will. The argument is wrong on two counts: (1) It confuses conscious and unconscious meanings; and (2) it confuses the primary and secondary gain of the illness.

The primary significance of symptom formation and character deviation is invariably the defense against instinctual impulses. The symptom is an inadequate compromise between drive and defense. The environment reacts to the symptom. For example: The concerned husband of the hysterical patient feels sorry for his wife, and makes efforts to comfort her, because she felt hurt out of all proportion when he had paid a compliment to her friend. This in no way signifies that the true motive of the patient's pouting and ill-humor was to draw attention to herself. The infantile attitude of the hysterical patient towards his environment not infrequently recapitulates the old emotional relationship to the mother. Freud has pointed out that the man hopes to inherit the girl's feelings towards her father, but instead he often finds that she expects him to play the role of the providing and indulgent mother.

Another aspect of infantile attitudes is related to excessive egocentricity. After this character deformation has become established, the people in the environment are used solely as suppliers of gratification. It has become impossible for the patient to consider the needs of others, to experience empathy and to identify with others. Hysterical persons inflict much pain on others through their egocentric lack of human concern. These patients not infrequently display a mixture of sentimentality and an unfeeling indifferent attitude. I know patients who have spent half of their vacation time grieving about a bird hit by their car, yet who are indifferent to the fact that in the course of time they have made many people very unhappy. The hysterical patient welcomes indulgence, he wants to be protected and treated like a nursery plant; he thinks that his attachment to people who treat him accordingly is love; on the basis of all these traits we are indeed entitled to designate him as egocentric. Perhaps one could also use the expression egoistic, but that word has a rather moralizing sound. Infantilism has led us to egocentricity. To be egocentric frequently also means to put oneself into the center of attention. The hysterical patient shares this trait with many neurotics. Because of the inhibition of their instinctual strivings and the high demands of their ego ideal they constantly take themselves as an object of reflection and meditation. Hysterical patients are inclined to think of their own traits and attitudes as the norm. They dwell on the peculiarities of their character as if they were matters of world-shaking importance. Not what they are and experience is the important issue, but that they experience, that they feel one way or another. They consider themselves an amazing phenomenon. They are indeed a source of wonder for the psychiatrist. The observer who is not fascinated by these patients on the basis of his own neurosis perceives their reactions as stereotyped and therefore frustrating and disappointing. Similarly, many people in their environment admire these personalities, while others view them with very little sympathy. Our knowledge informs us that only through psychotherapy can these persons be helped to develop genuine feelings and empathy with other human beings. It would be erroneous to assume that these patients are unable to have genuine feelings; they can be taught to experience them. It is very moving to observe in the course of a successful psychotherapy the development of profound, genuine emotions and of concerned relationships with others. Even the apparently radiant hysterical patients who impress others because of their intense need to elicit admiration are aware of the absence of true human relationships; their hidden wounds are painful in spite of the glittering façade. A hysterical patient expressed this in the phrase, "I have no character; I am empty." The degree of suffering of these patients is very impressive, and many observers tend to pay more attention to this suffering than to the pain that the patients inflict on others. One's reaction to hysterical patients depends on the circumstances of the mutual relationship. In everyday life one will have to deal with their behavior and its consequences and will not deny that the patients fail in their relationships to others. At the same time the physician and the psychologist have to concern themselves with the unconscious conflicts which motivate the patient's behavior.

We must still discuss the last member of the triad, the lack of genuineness (Kuiper, 1958). This refers mainly to expressions of emotions, even though the emotions themselves can be spurious. It was once assumed that the spuriousness of emotional manifestations was the result of an organic cerebral defect, localized in the areas of the brain related to emotional life. A thorough phenomenological investigation shows that such as assumption is not tenable. The patient with spu-

rious feelings is compelled to assume a certain attitude because of unconscious motivations. He perceives this attitude
as the proper and accepted one, both in the view of his environment and his conscience. The essential motive is the patient's fear of being rejected and condemned. Connected
with it is the fear of his own instinctual impulses, because
their emergence into consciousness and their pressing toward
action calls forth unbearable feelings of guilt. We must
elaborate on our statement that the patient is compelled to
assume a certain attitude. Spurious emotions seem to be so
much a part of the patient's personality that one hesitates to
call them pathological. Is not this attitude the result of a certain constitutional predisposition? A quality like this is not
only external. Zutt (1929) has contributed a significant essay
on the "internal attitude." We demonstrated the great importance of the postulate of an internal attitude for the
expression of emotions. Let us imagine the following situation. Someone has suffered a loss, and wants to conceal his
grief. He does not have to decide at every moment how to
conduct himself. In certain situations he will not express his
sorrow; he will act as if it were no matter, he will assume an
inner attitude of someone who goes about his daily tasks as
if nothing extraordinary has happened. However, when he
meets a friend, he can assume an attitude which corresponds
to his sorrow. The inner attitude determines the expression of
emotions.

In my search for a psychological explanation of spuriousness I was struck by the observation that some people are
spurious only in definite situations. I mention a woman who,
married to an artist, demands of herself that she not only
speak the artists' language but also experience and display
the artists' emotions. This does not, however, fit her own
style at all. As soon as such a person senses that she is respected and liked by her husband's friends (even though she
abstains from making profound statements about realistic and

abstract paintings), that she is being accepted for herself, her spuriousness disappears. One can speak of situational spuriousness, which occurs when the patient is anxious lest he be rejected. But when the fear of being rejected is not related to a situation in reality, when instead, an agency within the patient approves of only one specific inner posture, then habitual spuriousness develops. The agencies in question, the superego and ego ideal, are formed on the basis of parental attitudes. Parents prescribe not only certain rules of conduct, they also expect the children to have certain feelings. To do good is not sufficient, to be good is the demand. When the demands are too high and the child cannot meet them with his own resources, he still assumes the attitude demanded by the parents. Not only does he behave like a good child, he pretends to feel like one; he intensely wants to experience himself as good and to feel the appropriate emotions.

Aldous Huxley pointed out in a paper about situational and habitual spuriousness read at the Menninger Clinic that this spuriousness is very much determined by social and cultural factors. Often the demand is made of us to be what we are not. Spuriousness will occur quite frequently in the presence of a strict conscience. When the possibility of a genuine relationship is blocked because of an intense inhibition of the sexual life, and the pressure towards gratification is nevertheless very strong, the approach to another human being will be made in a spurious manner. There are ungenuine feelings in all areas of experience. There are also spurious expressions of passion. Spuriousness is a result of unsuccessful imitation in response to cultural and social pressures. Once in operation, it exerts an influence on the culture. Many people no longer seem capable of distinguishing between genuine and nongenuine emotions. The categories true and false are much too seldom applied by the art critics, although their use clarifies much, and would contribute to the education of the public. This in turn, would make it easier to educate children in this respect. Thus concepts emanating from the theory of the neuroses are applicable in many areas of human endeavor; they are certainly helpful in understanding the social and cultural phenomena which contribute to the formation of the neuroses.

In my opinion psychiatric literature pays too little attention to the masochistic aspect of the hysterical character, often one of its very pronounced traits. The term masochism has multiple meanings. In the broadest sense masochism is the wish to suffer pain, grief and humiliation. This wish can be conscious (as in the masochistic perversion in which pain is accompanied by sensual pleasure.) Or unconscious (when no conscious pleasure in pain is experienced and one unconsciously exposes oneself to grief, to assuage guilt and to satisfy a need for punishment). In the latter instance, we refer to moral masochism, indicating the participation of a conflict of conscience. A severe, even sadistic superego imposes punishment on the ego. The ego submits to it in order to be relieved from an unbearable feeling of guilt. The hysterical patient shows aspects of both forms of masochism. The patients' intense feelings of guilt generate a need for punishment, and compel a continuous search for atonement. All pleasure is prohibited to them, they must lose life's promising chances, and all success must be turned into failure. The sexual form of masochism is also present, though it usually is more or less disguised. The wish to have surgical operations is often the expression of a masochistic sexual fantasy in which a powerful man takes pity on the helpless body. If one is familiar with the relationship between hysteria and sexual repression it is not surprising that many abdominal operations are consequences of hysterical complaints. The feelings of hysterical patients towards their physician are indeed often "erotized." Only in this form is the relationship with a man permitted: "I need him for the treatment of my illness."

There are neurotic conditions in which moral masochism occupies a central position. These characters are burdened by deep feelings of guilt, they are constant victims of misfortune and unhappiness, against which they forever protest in vain.

OBSERVATIONS ON THE DEPTH PSYCHOLOGY OF THE HYSTERICAL NEUROSES

The preceding discussion leads us to attempt a depth psychological interpretation of hysteria and the hysterical character. A phenomenology that is not content with a superficial description of perceptions, and does not degenerate into a play with words, is bound to encounter the manifestations and connections to which attention has been called by psychoanalytically oriented investigators. A comprehensive psychoanalytic interpretation of the hysterical neuroses far exceeds the scope of this primarily clinically oriented chapter. I refer the reader to the professional literature, mainly to Freud's works on hysteria, and Otto Fenichel's (1945) book, *The Psychoanalytic Theory of the Neuroses.*

Symptoms and character deformations are a consequence of the inhibition of the sexual and aggressive instinctual drives. Hysterical patients succumb to the usual societal prohibitions against drives, failing to integrate their sexual and aggressive needs into their personality. Inadequate educational measures are responsible for this state of affairs, and the perpetuation of these measures is its fateful consequence. Man does not follow here the Aristotelian principle that the drive can and must be integrated, but perceives the drives as the result of the soul's imprisonment in the body, or as a sign of the fall of man. This attitude of the educator frustrates the children and forces them to renounce instinctual gratifications; as a consequence thereof the drives remain fixated on an infantile developmental level, and the growing child never learns to reasonably manage his instinctual strivings.

In the presence of certain constitutional predispositions and unfavorable environmental influences the hysterical neuroses develop in constant interaction between the individual and the environment. The normal developmental processes stagnate, the Oedipus complex is repressed instead of being resolved. These very general remarks naturally give no account of the way in which the individual development is disturbed in a particular case.

It is still a common view that psychoanalysts make one specific pathogenic factor responsible for the neurosis, for instance a psychic trauma like the seduction of a little boy by the maid, sexual games, or the child's observation of a sexual act between grown-ups, etc. Freud discovered that many reports of seduction are based not on reality but on the child's fantasies. Nevertheless, these fantasies can have a pathogenic effect. At present much emphasis is put on unfavorable traumatic situations rather than single traumatic events. In such situations, or in reaction to them, the child develops fantasies which become pathogenic because they cannot be openly expressed, and are instead repressed. Paternal prohibitions and the commands of the developing superego share in the responsibility for the necessity of repression; in addition certain intrapsychic conflicts, such as those between aggression and libido and between active and passive strivings provide the impetus for repression. All this does not completely invalidate the traumatic theory of the neurosis. There are many detrimental circumstances which make the child vulnerable, and an event can thus have a pathogenic effect on him, while another less vulnerable child will master a similar experience with relative ease. Thus a boy who was brought up with puritanical strictness and has many guilt fantasies will react very strongly to a castration threat, or to an urgent infantile instinctual impulse. It is possible that the development of excessively intense sexual ties to the parents is favored by the strictness of the prohibition of all erotic interests and all sexual advances of children to one another. Thus a particularly powerful Oedipus complex in the genital phase is conditioned by the preceding stages of development. Once established, the oedipal conflicts provide an etiological factor for later neurotic disturbances.

The prohibitions of the oedipal period retain their effect throughout the life of the patient suffering from a hysterical neurosis. The repressed drives find their expression and occasionally their gratifications in conversion symptoms. In this way some discharge of drive energies is possible, since the conscience is "paid off" by the admixture of considerable suffering to the pleasure. At the same time the repressed sexual and aggressive impulses continue their thrust towards consciousness, as can be seen from the anxiety which is so common a symptom in hysteria. The previously mentioned examples of the appearance of anxiety in the course of psychoanalytic treatment can be understood as incidents of psychic trauma resulting in intense anxiety. Conditions with disturbed consciousness tend to favor dramatization of conflicts.

The investigation of the hysterical neuroses began with the study of the drive and its disturbances. At present much attention is paid to the operation of conscience and to the disturbances of the ego functions. It is not too speculative to think of these disturbances in terms of an inappropriate use of energy. The energy required for the defense against infantile instinctual impulses is withdrawn from the integrating function of the ego and from adaptation.

Frigidity and impotence are nuclear symptoms of the hysterical neuroses. Sexuality remains attached to infantile positions, and old prohibitions are still in force; all this is expressed in disturbances of the sexual functions. Hysterical character traits are not to be regarded as immutable, constitutionally determined features. The infantile nature of the hysterical character represents a developmental disturbance.

We have also called attention in detail to hysterical egocentricity, the misuse of interpersonal relationships for narcissistic purposes and the scanty capacity for empathy.

It requires no metaphysical or constitutional interpretation to understand and explain the spuriousness of the hysterical person's emotions. When genuine feelings are lacking because of the neurotic disturbance of development, when emotions rooted in instinctual needs are absent because of repression and the patients feel compelled at the same time to demonstrate certain affects, they assume an "inner attitude" which is at odds with the rest of their personality.

4

∞∞∞∞◊◊∞∞∞◊

HYSTERICAL NEUROSES
IN FEMALES

THE FIXATION to the oedipal stage of development is central to the pathogenesis of the classical hysterical neuroses. In order to escape from the difficulties of the oedipal phase, some patients retreat to earlier stages of development. They ward off their problems through regression. Regression leads to formation of different symptoms in boys and in girls, hence we have to discuss them separately. The symptoms and character deformations of women have their main origin in the castration complex; those of men originate in the so-called negative Oedipus complex. A clinical classification is impossible without considering the psychogenesis of the symptoms. The genetic reflections of the psychoanalytic theory enabled us to delineate and to understand these conditions. I shall endeavor to stress the clinical and descriptive aspects. Let us begin with the neuroses of the female.

NEUROTIC REACTIONS TO
THE CASTRATION COMPLEX

We have already mentioned that in the course of her development the little girl goes through a phase of jealousy of the little boy. Some psychiatrists regard penis envy as a normal phenomenon and see the decisive pathogenic factor in quantitative differences. It is also possible to consider penis envy as such as a pathological phenomenon. In my opinion, broad empirical investigations are required before a final answer to this question can be given. Psychoanalytic theory ascribes to penis envy a change in the child's attitude to her parents, and describes some consequences of that change. The girl is angry at her mother, an all-powerful figure in the child's mind, for withholding from the child the organ possessed by boys. She turns her emotions to the father who has not inflicted this injustice on her, and who moreover is in possession of the passionately desired organ. Lampl-de Groot (1927) was the first to point out that the little girl goes through a phallic phase. In this phase she displays much similarity to the boy. Thus Lampl-de Groot made a discovery of fundamental significance for our insight into female psychology. In agreement with Helene Deutsch, Freud (1931, 1933) emphasized the feelings of hostility towards the mother in this phase.

We shall bear in mind two points in regard to the psychopathology of the neuroses in women: (1) Jealousy of the man plays a decisive role for the formation of most neurotic disorders of the woman. (2) Female neurotic patients have a hostile attitude to their mothers, sometimes hidden and sometimes quite open. This hostility has its foundation in the castration complex and in oedipal jealousy.

It is disastrous for the development of the little girl if the parents let her know that they really wanted a boy. In such a situation the penis envy receives powerful stimulation. The attitude "we would have preferred a boy" disturbs the relationship to the mother most of all. Moreover, the latter not uncommonly feels inadequate because she could not bear a son for her husband. The mother's discontent is often given vent in the relationship to her little daughter. If the father subsequently also rejects the little girl we have a very neurosogenic situation before us. The child feels insecure in her

relationship to both parents. In this setting both the preoedipal and oedipal situations are pathogenetic. All relationships
to people in later life tend to be disturbed by jealousy,
hatred, feelings of inferiority and general discontent with
herself and others. Hidden deeply underneath all that is a
profound longing for security, a security impossible of attain-
ment, because the neurosis disturbs the very relationships in
which a normal person feels secure and sheltered, such as a
love relationship, or a happy marriage. The relationship to
the man is disturbed through neurotic regression to the phallic phase. Vehement reactions of jealousy are the consequence. Regression to the still earlier oral phase takes these
patients into an extremely dependent relationship characterized by an insatiable need for love. This deep regression
often raises the ambivalence of the emotions immensely. Abraham (1920), has in his classical monograph, "Manifestations
of the Female Castration Complex," described two forms of
reaction to the castration complex. He named them the
wish-fulfillment type and the revenge type. Thus there are
women who deny the sex difference by assuming a posture
which says "I can do everything better than the man." Others use their feminine qualities and attributes to render the
man helpless. In this manner they take their revenge for the
presumed injustice inflicted on them.

I can imagine that the reader expects at this point to hear
of the domineering and castrating female. However, I should
like to caution against a careless use of these terms, not because they are used pejoratively by some but because these
concepts have too many meanings and therefore are all too
easily misunderstood. The lay public has appropriated these
terms and uses them indiscriminately. Men who find themselves defeated in a discussion by a woman of superior intelligence don't hestitate to call her domineering. The inept and
inhibited man who feels sexually rejected by a woman, because she occasionally wants to engage in a conversation and

not only in sexual intercourse, takes revenge by referring to her as a castrating female.

Female colleagues who have not properly adapted in their role as wife and mother commit the analogous error. The first thing they discover about a man is his phallic-narcissistic behavior or his latent homosexuality. It is always advisable to be aware of one's own psychic bias and to guard against the distortion of one's perception. Acquisition of scientific foundations is part of psychiatric training. Usually a training analysis is required to eliminate one's psychic blind spots.

After these cautionary words let us turn to the types described by Abraham (1920):

The wish-fulfillment type of woman indicates by words and behavior that she can do everything a man can do. The belief in the truth of this statement is not pathological. Why should a woman not be able to do what a man can? Very few accomplishments are indeed not within her power. For example, we know female politicians, scientists, artists, athletes of world renown, etc. The protests of men against women's participation in "all male" endeavors often represent an attempt to hold on to the feeling of male superiority that requires for its support the assumption of women's limitations. The fact that a woman excels in male activities is not neurotic, but when the wish to excel acquires the quality of an addiction, we deal with a neurotic reaction. The wish-fulfillment type also has revenge needs; the wish is not only to excel, but also to belittle and humiliate the man.

How can we distinguish between a normal attitude toward work and a neurotically competitive urge, when the contemporary social and cultural influences encourage the woman to play a role in life so very different from the role she was expected to play in the past? In the neurotic woman, intense hostility towards the man accompanies the need to achieve. She cannot collaborate with the man, begrudges him his success, is excessively and unfairly critical, and tends to stir up strife between men. We can add, such a woman will fail in a situation which requires specifically feminine behavior. She is unable to receive passively, she is frigid and will conceal this frigidity by avoiding all situations in which her sexual inadequacy could become evident. These traits have often been ascribed to a masculine constitutional factor. Such a factor may occasionally play a contributing role; however, every psychotherapist with some experience is familiar with the attractive, well-dressed, elegant woman who before therapy was a masculine, crudely attired patient. Sometimes hysterical symptoms are also to be found in such cases, but the character neurosis and the interpersonal disturbances are definitely predominating. Of special interest are the neurotic relationships which these women eventually develop with their marriage partners. These relationships determine the milieu in which the children are reared, often with conspicuously detrimental results.

The woman with the classical hysterical syndrome often marries a man who is given to rescue fantasies. The "sensitive" girl, attracted by the "gentle" man expects that he will not make her miserable with "that terrible sexuality," using sex only as a means for procreation.

The woman of the wish-fulfillment type tends to marry a man who was reared by a dominating mother and continues a similar relationship in the marriage. He is very dependent on her, she determines the way his earnings are spent, the number of children and their education and also his "ration" of sexual gratification, which she grants him as reward for his submissive behavior. When the man fails to subordinate himself to her wishes he is punished by withholding of sexual favors. Such a behavior pattern must be regarded as pathological. It is not sufficient to speak of a tyrannical character trait; the psychiatrist has to pay attention to the neurotic suffering, even though it may be quite effectively concealed. The domineering attitude of the woman is underscored when she is disappointed by the unmanly conduct of her spouse. If the man behaves in a masculine manner and not like a dependent child, even the domineering woman can permit herself the emergence and gratification of her invariably present feminine wishes. Shakespeare's *The Taming of the Shrew* demonstrates how a peremptory, hot-tempered girl can be brought to submission. As a rule, the measures used in Shakespeare's comedy do not suffice in life; in most cases only psychotherapy helps.

In a neurotic marriage relationship the partners for the most part do not feel in need of help. The partners act out their neuroses in life, and satisfy their need to dominate and be dominated. The child psychiatrist sees these mothers in the child guidance centers; their children have neurotic disturbances generated in part by the mothers' inability to accept their female role. The boys were either forced into helpless dependence, or driven to seek impossible accomplishments. They are to win successes withheld from the mothers. The boys' sexuality is strictly suppressed. The girls suffer various neurotic difficulties based on the castration complex.

No less common is a different neurotic relationship between the woman of this type and her partner. The man is being used to dominate and impress others, the man acts in a sense as the aggressive male alter ego of these women. Glover aptly called the men in this situation the women's sadistic penis. The *cherchez la femme* gives us in such situations the answer to why certain men temporarily or even permanently behave in a peremptory manner, displaying a lust for power, and attributes which are foreign to their general character. The following serves to illustrate this: A business man who was regularly absent from his office for short periods of time, behaved upon his return in a strict manner with his employees, sharply criticizing them for their laxity. This was so well-known in his plant that no one dared to ask him for anything shortly after his return, postponing the request for a week or so when he became approachable again. He felt constantly threatened by his colleagues, and used to talk at length about the need for good cooperative efforts, etc. The *cherchez la femme* led to the discovery that he spent the days of absence from his business with his mistress in a neighboring town. This woman was herself a successful executive, much feared by her employees because of her arrogant and high-handed manner. She was said to be "wearing the pants" in her office. Our entrepreneur was the instrument used to act out her aggressive fantasies, which had their origin in the castration complex. Such women incite their men to "virile" aggressive behavior with a variety of critical arguments. Within the family such women urge the fathers to be particularly strict with the children. Experienced personnel managers are quite familiar with family situations of this nature. They know that in many cases the wives cause the difficulties of their employees; the wives accuse them of softness and urge them to be competitive and aggressive. Thus emerges the typical pattern of a man who is henpecked at home, and a pompous and harsh employer at work.

Du Boeuff pointed out that some hysterical patients actively turn to the environment while others withdraw from it. He spoke of active and passive hysteria. The patients who actively turn toward the world frequently possess the qualities of the wish-fulfillment type described above. I have already pointed out the necessity for a certain clinical classification, and have observed that the transitions between the neuroses are extraordinarily fluid. When the clinical differentiation is difficult the dynamic and genetic points of view can help us to clarify the matter. Classical hysteria and the hysterical character are rooted in the unresolved Oedipus complex. Because the castration complex is so important for the genesis of neuroses we have provided a special classification for the consequences of the castration complex; we place these neurotic sequelae of the penis envy in the category of phallic hysterical disorders. The concept of phallic hysteria is of advantage because it takes cognizance of its relatedness to the classical neurosis. There are, of course, transitional forms between the classical and the phallic neuroses. Inhibitions in the sexual area and penis envy are often interconnected. To evaluate a neurosis we must estimate the relative significance of the prohibition of heterosexual interests and of penis envy.

The course of a hysterical illness can be extraordinarily capricious. The symptoms change, as does their respective basis. It should never be forgotten that, as a rule, the woman's wish to be a man is deeply repressed and unconscious. Only in some actively homosexual women does it appear undisguised.

When infantile sexual impulses dominate the erotic life we speak of perversions. Since we have learned that perversions have a defensive function as well, we observe not only the differences but also the similarities between neurosis and perversion.

The Vengeful Type. The character neurosis of the so-called vengeful type also has its origins in the castration complex. As we have seen, some of the patients under the influence of an unresolved castration complex attempt to remedy the defect by equalling or surpassing the man in intellectual and other pursuits, or by ruling over him in work and marriage. Others, dominated by envy of his possession of the penis, attempt to weaken him and render him helpless. These two "solutions" of the castration complex suggest themselves as natural.

When one envies another person one can attempt to possess the object of one's envy, or one can strive to destroy it. The latter path is for many the easier to follow. Abraham calls the neurotic woman who reacts in this way, the revengeful type. She revenges herself on the man who possesses what she lacks. This revenge can be expressed openly or disguised; it can be conscious or unconscious. When the impulse is openly acted out .we can speak of an alloplastic reaction and diagnose a psychopathic personality; when the revenge impulse is repressed, and we observe only the results of the repression, the reaction is autoplastic, and we deal with a neurotic condition.

The psychopathic type is familiar to us as the "vamp." This character type expresses itself in a repetitive maneuver: A man is seduced and made helplessly dependent, upon which there follows a characteristic behavior pattern. The woman makes ever higher demands, she wants to be not only taken care of, but extravagantly indulged. When she has taken from the man all he has to give, she turns away from him in triumph, or finds other admirers to stir up his jealousy. Not infrequently men are driven to suicide by such a woman. They commit suicide out of utter despair, overwhelmed by paralyzing fears of abandonment. The feeling of being abandoned means not being able to function as a man; he is castrated. Men get into these dangerous situations in consequence of a typical behavioral maneuver. The woman constantly arouses the man's sexual desires, which she at first gratifies, but then abruptly thwarts. The use of the word vampire illustrates well the sucking and biting aspects of the behavior pattern of these patients. The female genital is used like a biting mouth; one is reminded in this connection of the vagina dentata fantasy. The oral-sadistic attitude is one of the determinants of this form of the female castration complex. The following fantasy of a patient of this type is very illuminating: She imagined that she deprived all the men she had or could have intercourse with of their penises, which she then strung on a line like trophies in her room. This type of woman is a rewarding subject in literature, on the stage and in films. As long as the partner, or better, the victim is in the process of being conquered, love is convincingly feigned; there are many nuances between deliberate feigning and feelings that lack genuineness.

The neurotic form of this vengeful type shows symptoms among which neurotic infidelity, the inability to commit oneself, is one of the most important symptoms. The vengeful and hostile attitude toward the man is unconscious, and the infatuation which introduces the maneuver is not feigned, or not even ungenuine; the infatuation can be particularly passionate. But to be capable of infatuation by no means implies that the person is also capable of loving. Rather, the infatuation is an expression of demand, a clamoring anticipation of wish-fulfillments. As soon as the partner is won, a curious phenomenon takes place, the woman begins to doubt her choice, she finds herself less and less attracted to the man. The vanishing of the infatuation is in some instances perceived as an ego-alien painful symptom. The patient experiences a fate worse than that of Tantalus from whose mouth the water receded when he tried to drink it; for the patient the water, once available, loses the very qualities which slake thirst. In the same moment in which the man declares his love, her love vanishes. Sometimes the infidelity has a narcissistic significance: "I am a person of such complexity, of such highly differentiated needs that no one man can satisfy all of them." In such cases the inability to love is not an ego-alien symptom, but an ego-syntonic character trait.

It is clear that such patients inflict much unhappiness on their partners. The man is won, then rejected and in a very real sense robbed of his virility, at least as long as he feels himself committed to the woman. How is their fixation to be explained? A precondition of so intense an attachment to a woman of the psychopathic vamp type reveals masochism in the man. In women of the neurotic revenge type the castration tendency is very deeply hidden and discernible only to the psychiatrist. The woman was in love and experiences the disappearance of her love as painful. This reaction continues to kindle her partner's feelings. Besides, she assures him that she will always remain his best friend, and what man fails to hear such assertions with pleasure and hopeful anticipation? He fails to realize that he remains in bondage to this woman, and plays the role of the heartbroken lover into which his castrating lady friend has cast him. He perceives only the sad result and is without comprehension of what is happening between them. These maneuvers remind one of the copulation of the praying mantis in the course of which the male is devoured by the female. Sometimes a woman who torments her man in this way herself suffers from her faithlessness and feels guilty about it. At times only a thin layer of pity conceals her triumphant feelings like a thin coat of sugar around a bitter pill. It is a grievous version of the love potion, which unlike the one in *Tristan and Isolde*, is taken by only one of the lovers.

The revenge is not always limited to the triumphant rejection of the lover. It is even more painful for the man to be made jealous by the woman's turning to another man. One woman of this reaction type always managed to send her lover away in the middle of the night so that she could spend the rest of it with the other man. She could not decide on a choice between the two men, believing she loved both equally well. On rare occasions suicide and homicide occur in consequence of such maneuvers. The man has been emasculated and the woman receives her punishment for the wish to castrate the man. Helene Deutsch pointed out that Carmen represents such a compulsively faithless woman, in the end she provokes her violent punishment. Sometimes the infatuation flares up when the man makes efforts to break off the relationship. It is characteristic for such affairs that only one partner at a time is certain that he or she is in love, and this occurs invariably when the other partner is uncertain and wavering in his feelings. The men experience the behavior of their lover as very mystifying.

It is easier to desire than to love. In our fantasy the other is always as we want him to be. His image does not necessarily resemble our own person, instead it is in accordance with our profoundest wishes. In fantasy, we readily idealize the beloved. Reality is always more or less disappointing. In order to love one must be able to bear frustrations. The person who cannot tolerate frustrations will not progress from being in love to true love. In the case of the castrating woman the discrepancy between desire and love is neurotically exaggerated, because the wish to castrate prevails over the wish to love. In some situations there is marginal adaptation, but usually the relationship ends disastrously because of the unchanging penis envy. Quantitative factors are of decisive significance. Some women like to win their man repeatedly, others are periodically preoccupied with fantasies of faithlessness. The representatives of this type of reaction turn the man down again and again. Often they finally marry a man whom they esteem less than some of their preceding lovers. Marriage to the least loved man is sometimes a punishment for the castrating tendency. Sometimes marriage is possible only with a man of moderate virility. As Abraham demonstrated in his excellent essay, these women cannot bear the proximity of masculine partners.

Many neurotic women are very inhibited. They are particularly attractive to some men, to whom they appear mysterious. As already stated, the men can project onto them a rich web of fantasy. For some men these women represent a kind of "superwoman," in analogy to the superman figure.

Originally the dynamic and genetic interpretation of the hysterical neuroses emphasized their origin in the Oedipus complex. But much of the hysterical patient's suffering will remain unintelligible if we do not also consider the intrapsychic tensions which result from conflicts between superego and ego ideal. There are cases of classical hysteria in which the ego ideal has joined the superego in condemning and prohibiting instinctual impulses. Women of this type display frank contempt for everything instinctual. They hold that these lowly matters are fitting only for "inferior" people. Other women of this type feel the same contempt, but strive to conceal it. If one directs questions to them about the matter, they reply: "You know, Doctor, the man needs that kind of thing." The low regard for the man is unmistakable. The intrapsychic conflicts are often complicated; the prohibiting, stern superego may be paired with an ego ideal which prescribes that the woman act as an ideal loving housewife to her husband. There is a double conflict situation between superego and drive, and superego and ego ideal. The instinctual impulses required for the satisfaction of the demands of the ego ideal cannot be gratified, one cannot be simultaneously a loving wife and, in obedience to the superego, a frigid woman—or at most, only to a very small degree. Obviously, a sexual attitude demanded by the ego ideal but impossible because of superego restrictions will lead to the development of spurious feelings. A patient perceived herself in her fantasies as the wife of a man to whom she attached herself and then triumphantly sent away. Yet she also saw herself as the mother of his children. This is how she described her conscious intentions, "To be a companion, to have a lovely family, and to bring up the children along enlightened principles." In reality she made life so unhappy for her friend that he finally broke with her and married another young woman who had the same name as the patient. Her instinctual needs were approved by her ego ideal and motivated her to take up erotic relationships, but her castration complex constantly induced her to humiliate the man.

The woman with a neurotic variation of the revenge type wants to be loving fiancée intent on marriage, but the acting out of the castration complex and the need for revenge make this position untenable. The observable wish to be loved and to be wife and mother make the sudden change from the ideal beloved into a rejecting, scornful, cold beauty particularly incomprehensible for the man.

The discrepancy between wish and incapacity to enact it is common to other areas of life as well. Our society expects its daughters to grow up to be loving wives. But development of a healthy sexual life necessary for that purpose is impeded or prevented by unreasonable prohibitions and by secrecy, which in itself has the effect of a prohibition. Again, reasonable methods of child rearing could have a prophylactic effect and spare us much grief.

The direction of neurotic development is to some degree codetermined by the personality's endowment. The investigation of the disturbed adaptation must include the study of the personality's gifts and abilities, its potential, i.e., the qualities which belong to the autonomous functions of the ego, Hartmann (1939). I was struck by the large number of women of the revenge type who are intellectually inferior and emotionally barren. I shall mention one example: A high official was unhappy in his marriage and began an affair with a woman towards whom he felt a very strong sexual attraction. He contemplated marrying her. She was occasionally unfaithful, but that made her still more desirable to him. With conspicuous naïveté he argued that a woman wanted by others must be particularly desirable. In addition to her infidelity this woman was also uneducated and had no meaningful interests in life. Her stupidity could not entirely be explained by lack of education and interests. Half in scorn, half in disappointment he described her to a friend as his most stupid mistress. As time went along he began to regard her stupidity and faithlessness as burdensome, as an impediment not compensated for by the sexual gratification. The relationship came to an end. I believe that the development of the neurosis of a number of women of this type is facilitated by a lack of possibilities in many areas of reality, and that they search for compensation in one specific area. The trite, yet important unconscious motive could be expressed as follows: "Even though I can accomplish nothing worthwhile,

I am still a very attractive woman, I shall make the most of it." Naturally the lack of ability does not cause the neurosis, which has its roots in the castration complex, but it accentuates this particular neurotic reaction, especially when owing to her physical beauty the woman has some chances for success in her sexual and erotic life. She becomes aware of it through the behavior of the men around her. Each new amorous experience strengthens her belief in her irresistibility. I believe that many women of the revenge type respond in this particular way to their castration complex because they are not gifted enough to compete with men on an intellectual level or on other levels. Our observation again confirms the statement that our endowment determines what we do with our neurotic problems, and these problems determine what we can accomplish with our artistic or intellectual endowment.

The intelligence and intellectual performance of women of the wish-fulfillment type receives particular stimulation from the fact that these functions are used in the service of neurotic adaptation.

CASTRATING THROUGH LOVE

Among the favorite and frequently used concepts of psychiatrists, psychologists and social workers are the expressions "dominating through love," and "castrating through love." Although these terms are more descriptive than the terms "psychopathic" or "hysterical" some caution in their use appears advisable.

A loving, domineering mother never lets her children grow up. She stifles their development by her exaggerated concern for her child. "Mother knows best" is the typical attitude. It undermines the child's self-confidence and greatly impedes his independence. These mothers mean well, consciously they want nothing but the best for their children. However, the need to keep the children dependent is only thinly disguised by this attitude. It is very difficult for the child to assert himself in the face of so much loving concern, and guilt feelings burden his independent striving. Thus one can observe grown men watch their mother's face like an anxious dog watches his master. Because of this anxiety and their guilt feelings these men are incapable of going their own way. Under pressure of feeling mother means well, all their aggressive impulses are turned inward.

There are marriages in which the relationship between the spouses resembles greatly that between the lovingly domineering mother and her son. The man is being indulged but he must pay for it with the loss of his freedom. The concept castrate can be used in this context with some justification, because to deprive a man of his independence means to emasculate him.

An entirely different connection between love and castration is characteristic for the woman who can fall in love with a man but cannot bind herself to him. An example will explain what is meant better than a long theoretical discourse: A woman had an affair with a man who loved her dearly, but she turned him down when he asked her to marry him. She then became engaged to another man. The first man was unhappy for a long time but finally he succeeded in freeing himself from his attachment. He was able to mobilize enough will power to avoid meeting his former mistress, though she was quite willing to see him. One day she unexpectedly came to tell him that she was going to be married the next day: "I did not want to marry without speaking to you once more, I have to tell you that my feelings for you were sincere, there will always be a place for you in my heart. It is too bad that you cannot come to the church tomorrow. Shall I ever have an opportunity to show you my children? They will have the beautiful brown eyes of X (her future husband)."

The woman and her friend are likely to think of this speech as a sign of affection and interest, but examination of its result and conscious intent reveals this conduct as a form of castrating through love. The profession of affection serves the purpose of binding the man and blocking his way to another woman. The old fantasy of castration is transferred to the present situation. The woman does what she wanted to do as a little girl: she gets hold of the object for which she had envied the little boy and attempts to hold on to it.

In the foregoing we have described two forms of castration through love. The first can also be described as dominating through love.

FANTASIES OF RAPE AND PROSTITUTION

Neurotic manifestations like phobias, excessive modesty, inhibitions and a tendency to blush are often based on fantasies of rape and prostitution. Such fantasies can be more or less conscious or unconscious. The fantasy of being raped is a remarkable phenomenon, it is a typical example of "pleasure without guilt." The woman can assuage her guilt feelings about sexual gratification with the claim that she cannot be held responsible for what has happened, she was a victim, not an active participant in the experience. The study of rape fantasies can also provide a contribution for our understanding of racial hatred. Warded-off pleasurable fantasies about virility, unusually developed sexual organs, and the wish to be sexually attacked may result in protective hatred.

Fantasies of being raped have in common the components of a crude, initial approach by the man, tearing of the clothes, violent spreading of the legs and uncovering of the genitalia. The locale of the attack is usually the open street or the forest. Sometimes other men look on and then take turns in the rape; not infrequently the fantasy then sees them fighting each other and attempting to tear each other's penis off. It is not difficult to recognize here the contribution of the castration complex.

The wish for revenge plays a large part in the prostitution fantasies. While the rape fantasies with their "masochistic pleasure without guilt" are motivated by feelings of guilt about sexuality, and represent a compromise between wish and prohibition, sexual intercourse is forced upon one and it is painful. The prostitution fantasies focus on the wish to humiliate the man, to rob him of something, and also to make him jealous. It is not uncommon in such a fantasy that crowds of men line up before the girl's door and they fight each other for her favors. One of the aims of the fantasy can be described with these words: "I am not dependent on you, but you on me; I am not passive, but you are." Women of the psychopathic type act out such fantasies; in neurotic women the fantasies become the basis for the formation of neurotic symptoms, such as the fear of streets and other open places.

5

HYSTERICAL NEUROSES
IN MALES

THE DIFFERENCES in the psychosexual development between
men and women are so great that the corresponding hysterical neuroses have to be treated separately.

In regard to the classification the following may be stated:
We find in men the classical hysterical character, its psychopathic variant, and the inhibited reaction type. There also
occurs the phallic-narcissistic type, which we call the Don
Juan type, and a variant of the latter, the Don Juan of
success.

Of paramount importance for many neurotic characters
are their passive-feminine needs. For that reason we include
the discussion of homosexuality in this chapter, although this
problem is counted among the perversions. Without insight
into the significance of passive-feminine strivings for the
symptomatology one is in the dark and cannot comprehend
the character types to be dealt with here. We shall deal with
characters whose central conflict revolves around work disturbances, authority and masochistic needs. As in disucussing
the female hysterias we shall endeavor to give a dynamic,
genetic and developmental description.

One observes men with classical hysterical symptoms: conversion, anxiety, disturbances of consciousness, and the char-

acter traits of infantilism, masochism and nongenuineness. The lack of genuineness in the character is different in the man than in the woman. Spurious feelings of men often relate to cultural undertakings. While the egocentricity of hysterical women manifests itself in the search for narcissistic satisfaction and in the area of sexual experiences, the hysterical male expresses his need to assert his importance in affecting a differentiated emotional and intellectual inner life, artistic gifts and ethical concerns. Thus one is not surprised to read in a play written by a hysterical patient abundant expressions like "the profoundest tragedy of human experience." The generous use of sentimentality plays on the reader's emotions, yet it is obvious that the author lacks true capacity for empathy with others.

When the need to bolster one's importance is acted out in the realm of society, and power and influence are desired above all, an open and honest struggle for one's ideals is little in evidence. There is rather an effort to dominate people by means of slander and intrigue and to use them for one's own purposes. One correctly says about such people that they believe in nothing and no one but themselves. Generous use of spurious feelings is made by them in pursuit of their goals. Patients of this type are so destructive of others that one tends to forget that they are sick people. Their insincere feelings express themselves at times in baseless excitement and in vehement moral indignation in connection with events which an ordinary person faces soberly and quietly. For example, a hysterical patient of this type became extremely agitated about a trivial overcharge, as if a great crime had been committed against him. To this group of patients belong many snobbish people with cultural pretensions who claim to find nothing worthwhile in every day life.

Like the analogous conditions of the woman, the hysterical conditions of the man are based on an inhibition of heterosexual needs and on the inability to function as an independent and mature person. Our culture provides a fertile soil for the hysterical person. Representatives of the psychopathic types of hysteria are those men who are fixated on the level of the Oedipus struggle with the father, and strive for a single goal in life, to achieve esteem, fame, and power. Just as the female counterpart of this type is happy only when she is admired as the most beautiful of women, so these men are content only when they dominate other men. Their knowledge and skill have the same function as the jewels of the prima donna, namely, to attract attention and to occupy the center of the stage. They change their convictions in keeping with the taste of their public, and use dexterity and brutality to achieve their ends.

Their inability to identify with their victims makes it easy for them to use intrigue and slander to remove others from their path. The astute psychologist recognizes in their idealistic pronouncements and their tendency to preach morality to those who are helpless the telltale marks of persons who conceal their aggressive and sadistic inclinations from themselves. These patients think of themselves as the rescuers of mankind, an opinion not shared by those who know them. However, the life of these people is not without pain and suffering. They are lonely and forever in flight from their discontent. Their infantile sexuality attracts women with an unresolved castration complex who use them to satisfy their own need to dominate the man. Their striving for some kind of superior position is the continuation of the oedipal struggle. They never realize how much they pass by in life. We have described the psychopathic variant of this type, characterized by acting out and poverty of emotions, which is disguised by display of spurious feelings. This type is known in the psychiatric literature as the hysterical psychopath. It is easier to consider as patients people who suffer rather than those who primarily inflict suffering on others. Objective investigation reveals that the latter are no less in need of treatment than the inhibited hysterical patients. All manifestations of hysterical neurosis mentioned earlier also occur in male patients. Disturbances in men which originate in the positive Oedipus complex show much conformity with analogous symptoms of hysteria in women.

CHARACTER TRAITS

The character which forms the background for the symptoms is either the classical hysterical or the inhibited character. Symptoms based on feelings of guilt or on inhibition of heterosexuality are conspicuously in the foreground. The difficulties in the choice of a partner and the inhibition of heterosexual expression often result in a persistence of masturbation beyond the age in which it normally occurs. The problems of the struggle with masturbation are dealt with in a neurotic manner, and provide the foundations for feelings of guilt, which in turn lead to depressive hypochondriacal and/or paranoid reactions. For example:

A young man recently engaged seeks the help of a psychiatrist because he blushes violently whenever the lecturer approaches a sexual topic. He imagines that his classmates on observing his discomfort conclude that he was still masturbating and was unable to take his girl to bed. This erythrophobia sharply limited his social mobility. Another patient sought advice because he could not speak freely in many situations and felt that he would never find the right words. He felt very despondent. He dared not address the girls in the office, but he found a young woman in a restaurant with whom he felt less ashamed of himself, and with whom he eventually began an affair. She was employed as a maid. The frequent sexual experiences with her did not satisfy him, because there was no other common ground between them.

The conditions described here are often complicated by problems of passivity, to which we shall return in detail at a later time.

The unsuccessful resolution of the Oedipus complex can lead to other compromise solutions as well. One of them is manifest or repressed active homosexuality. When the little boy is strongly attached to his mother and, owing to her attitude, becomes very anxious about all sexual feelings, the result is often an identification with the mother. In future he will treat younger boys as he wished to be treated by his mother. That is a general psychic mechanism. A child gives to the doll what he or she has received or wished to receive from his mother. A woman pampers her little dog and experiences the loving care as if she had received it herself.

Many people avail themselves of this psychic mechanism in a sublimated form. It need not be a disturbing feature in their life. The man who cannot permit himself a solicitous, motherly attitude is restricted in his emotional life, but not further disturbed by it. However, the sexualized forms of the maternal attitudes are in many ways not without danger. Groups of people are often agitated by rumors and reports of homosexual behavior, and one hears questions like this one: "How is it possible that a respectable man, the head of a nice family, jeopardizes his position, his work and the future of his family by homosexual affairs?"

It is not too well known that along with the heterosexual attitude a homosexual position also occurs. It rests on a misidentification, i.e., an identification with the mother instead of with the father or a male father substitute. Such homosexual inclinations are a potential threat to men who have to deal with adolescents and young men. Adolescent boys are a particular source of temptation for men with intense latent homosexual traits. The combination of girlish and boyish adolescent features makes the adolescent boy an object of their intense desire. It frequently occurs that a teacher, a doctor, a youth counselor or psychologist succumbs to the temptation. The consequences are often equally disastrous for the seducer and the seduced. It means the end of his career for the former, and a decisive step towards a homosexual development for the latter.

There are various causes and motives for this particular expression of homosexuality. This sexual deviation is despised in our society. It is accompanied by so much inner conflict that human beings with homosexual inclinations find it hard to find a homosexual relationship which is relatively free of potential disaster, and which will not lead to serious consequences. The controlled or repressed impulses are forever striving for an outlet. A medical examination presents temptations for a doctor with homosexual inclinations. The insecure persons among the examiners take advantage of this situation because they lack the courage to seek a partner of the same sex in nonprofessional situations. The need for punishment plays an important role, too. The seduction of a minor, if discovered, carries with it heavy penalties.

For some patients only the child or the adolescent is the object of desire. The patients wish to do the same things for or to the adolescent, which they longed for in their childhood or adolescence. It is extraordinarily regrettable that so many patients with such problems turn to the specialist familiar with their abnormality only after the judge compels them to seek psychiatric treatment, and after much unhappiness has already occurred. Sometimes the patient has already consulted a psychiatrist. All too often the case is diagnosed without dynamic and genetic investigation, but such investigation is the only way to understand the problem and offer help. The possibilities for help have remained relatively unknown because psychoanalytic knowledge has been rejected for so long by official psychology, medicine and pedagogy. Sometimes substantial help can be given these patients, and sometimes it is possible to induce the patient not to act out his impulses in a dangerous and potentially diastrous manner. The patients are by no means always psychopathic, on the contrary, many are typically neurotic people. This is a tremendous problem for those concerned with the mental health of the general population. Every person struggling with the problem of homosexuality needs help. Candid discussion, understanding and insight must take the place of taboos and denials.

If we define hysteria as a neurosis which is connected with a fixation to, and an unsuccessful working through of the Oedipus complex, then active homosexuality belongs in the same category. However, it appears more appropriate to limit the concept of hysteria to its classical clinical picture. Acted out, homosexuality can be classified among the perversions. The antithesis perversion-hysteria is not absolute, since perversion too has a defensive function. In active homosexuality the disappointed love for the mother is warded off. Among mothers of homosexual patients the number of those who have blocked their sons' path towards heterosexuality is notable and it is further remarkable that many representatives of the women of the castrating type are to be found among them.

Along with the misidentification with the mother which follows disappointment of the feelings forming a part of the positive Oedipus complex, an additional etiological factor is of great moment and that is castration anxiety.

Girls and women arouse anxiety in many men because they unconsciously consider the absence of a penis the result of a mutilating injury, a castration wound. A sexual partner who does not arouse this anxiety is particularly desirable, i.e., one with a penis and no wound.

Frequently active homosexuality is complicated by its passive form. My intention is not to separate two sharply distinguished types of homosexuality, but rather to describe two patterns of a process which commonly occur in the same patient, though they may differ in their respective significance.

If one uses the patient's subjective experience as a reference point certain differences are evident. There is the man who in reality or in his fantasies approaches young boys and induces them to mutual masturbation or to some activity in which they take the passive role in the sexual act. Another man assumes the woman's passive role himself, and affects a feminine seductive manner. It would be a mistake to assume that the two types have nothing in common. There are similar processes in a varying degree operating in both men and the respective variations have to be worked out in therapy. Often the passive form is covered up by active homosexuality, passive behavior being unacceptable to the person's self-esteem. By way of identification with the partner one's own passive homosexual needs receive vicarious gratification. Many neurotic men at first report active homosexual fantasies, and only later one discovers quite pronounced passive-feminine attitudes as well. Finally it must be pointed out that homosexual fantasies are often used as escape from heterosexuality, and vice versa. It cannot be concluded that in such a case one deals with a perversion, and consequently the case has a dubious therapeutic prognosis. Such an assumption is particularly erroneous when one notes the presence of heterosexual inclinations along with the homosexual inclinations. In such cases, the fear of heterosexuality has to worked through first. Actually all homosexuality is one of necessity. It is activated because the access to heterosexuality is barred. The necessity is either the psychic inhibition of heterosexual activity, or external factors—e.g., homosexuality occurring in an exclusively male setting because of the absence of women. A thorough revision of sex education is a precondition for preventing homosexuality. Our education suppresses heterosexuality. School children are ridiculed when they fall in love, and the only advice which the adolescent hears is that he stay out of trouble. Instead of being attacked heterosexuality should be nurtured. Experience shows that the development towards mature heterosexuality is not simple or easy.

Man has to learn laboriously what animals discover without effort by instinct.

To the complications following in the wake of a positive Oedipus complex belongs the symptom of degradation of love life. Some men worship one woman from a distance but sexually desire another. With them, love and desire do not synthesize, but remain mutually exclusive.

Inhibition of the sexual life appears clearly in the personality's response to the masturbation of adolescence. Exaggerated feelings of guilt, general discontent, and depressive reactions are common. Fear of organic disease is also not unusual. ("Whoever is as bad as I am must be punished by illness.") It is only a short step from these ruminations to a hypochondriacal preoccupation, and finally, to a paranoid response, when the boy believes that persons in his environment recognize that he secretly indulges in gratifying his needs. These typical reactions to the masturbation of adolescence reappear again later in life whenever the integration of the personality is disturbed or dissolved. They also appear within the delusional system of the schizophrenic, albeit together with other symptoms of this psychosis.

Whether one includes the results of a general inhibition of sexuality among the hysterical manifestations is a question of terminology. It is very probable that this inhibition is connected with the Oedipus complex, the incest barrier and the castration anxiety related to it.

In our culture, adolescence seems to take place within a laboratory for experimental psychopathology. To generate neuroses all one has to do is to force people with strong drive impulses to employ excessively rigid defenses against the drive. This can be done through outspoken prohibitions, or the power of suggestion. This indeed happens quite often. Mine is not a pessimistic view; actually, it is optimistic, since it indicates the direction of preventive measures. After all, it was not a pessimistic attitude when physicians warned against drinking contaminated water.

THE NEGATIVE OEDIPUS COMPLEX

Like the hysterical woman the neurotic man can accept neither his own sexual role, nor his being an adult. His neurotic symptomatology has its roots in this fact.

When guilt feelings and castration fears are too intense the Oedipus complex cannot be resolved properly. The little boy no longer competes with his father, but submits to him and becomes too anxiety ridden to woo his mother. Even if he does not entirely turn his back on heterosexuality, he acquires a passive character; he develops fantasies about being affectionately stroked and petted. Along with the passive heterosexual strivings strong passive homosexual inclinations also develop. All this leads to the drives with passive aims gaining the upper hand: A submissive response to competitive situations develops. The submission becomes sexualized and thereby masochistic. It is this passive-feminine-masochistic position which forms the nuclear issue of many of the man's neurotic disturbances.

These problems are called by some the problems of passivity, a somewhat unclear designation since the term passivity has many meanings: e.g., it may mean insufficiently active, too feminine, or dependent like a child. In addition, one speaks of drives with passive aim, and also of the need for affection, for loving care, shelter and protection. All these are aspects of the negative Oedipus complex.

It is useful to review the human psychic development. The infant depends on others for his care, is rarely active, and receives his gratifications passively. His drives with a passive aim are thus gratified and provide pleasures beyond those obtainable later through activity.

The neurotic man uses the emotions of dependence and

affection which he experienced in the relationship with his mother to deny his positive Oedipus complex. He submits to the father, his dependence acquires a quasi-feminine character. The early infantile attachment to both parents is taken over by a passive-feminine attitude. Feminine and infantile traits as well as passivity are not neurotic as such. One must be passive to be able to receive. However, dependence and submission often become sexualized and used to ward off heterosexuality and healthy aggressivity. In that case there is a neurotic reaction. In short: passivity is essential for receptivity and thus for mental health; the sexualized masochistic forms of passivity are neurotic and disturb adaptation. An element of regression is also involved: A return to an attitude of early childhood in defense against an active pattern. One should never forget that even though one sees little of a manifest active conquering attitude, this does not mean that it is not present. It is not accessible because it is warded off, repressed and unconscious.

In some cases the passive-homosexual attitude is acted out. The mechanisms which we have described in active homosexuality are present in the passive form as well, but the essential factor in passive homosexuality is the regression to a submissive, dependent position. The inner experience and the behavior of these patients is determined by the castration anxiety. They are as obsessed with the male genitals as the female revenge type described earlier. The love of these patients for their partners is decidedly ambivalent and is more concerned with their physical male attributes than their personalities. Their intention is to reach their goal by way of submission, they want to receive and possess rather than give. These men can be termed castrating through love. Therein is to be found one of the reasons for the frequent lack of satisfaction in homosexual relations. Fenichel (1931) who has contributed significantly to our understanding of homosexuality calls this love the "apprentice's love," the love of the boy apprentice who would like to incorporate his master's power. The sublimated form of the passive attitude is of social significance. We are familiar with the man who submits to whomever is in power at the moment, and who is dominated by the unconscious wish to become that man's successor as rapidly as possible.

Though homosexuality plays an important role in many neurotic men, most of those who seek our help are not exclusively homosexual. Homosexual wishes occur in heterosexual people and induce many to seek medical advice. The occurrence of such wishes arouses anxiety, particularly when they occur at the time of a heterosexual contact, or when they emerge in the form of obsessive thoughts. Latent homosexuality leads to difficulties in the choice of a spouse, to neurotic infidelity and to pathological jealousy. Psychopathic personalities act out their latent homosexuality in promiscuity. The warded-off passive-feminine attitude plays a significant role in cases of work disturbances and authority conflicts. Quite frequently the latent homosexuality disturbs the interpersonal relationships. This occurs commonly when the passive needs are warded off by a pseudo masculine, boastful behavior, hardly a way to make friends.

Though it is difficult to align the neuroses which demonstrate the above described symptoms in a logical pattern we shall endeavor to do so.

Let us begin with the fear of being a homosexual in a man who has manifest bisexual inclinations. He reports as follows: "I am going with a girl, but I wonder whether I should marry her. I would dislike being without her, yet she means little to me. Sometimes I think of my friend and his girl, I imagine what they do together, we even sometimes talk about it. I am worried that I am really a homosexual. I have trouble at work, I am too restless, I cannot spend more than five minutes at my desk," etc. The social, cultural and religious milieu contributes to the factors which determine the kind of symptoms which develop in a given case. If such men attempt sexual intercourse before marriage they discover that they lack full sexual power. There is no complete gratification and no inner harmony. Sometimes hysterical conversions and other symptoms occur in the wake of attempts to establish a heterosexual relationship.

The following components contribute to homosexuality: identification with the mother, through the psychic mechanisms which we have described in active homosexuality; a sexualized, possibly masochistically tinged negative Oedipus complex; arrested development of the aggressive drive, with use of submission as defense against aggression in situations when some self-assertion would be a more adequate form of adaptation.

We still have to discuss the conflicts with authority, which give vent to many neurotic disturbances of male patients. For the most part the conflicts with authority have two aspects: First, the continuation of the oedipal rivalry with father figures in later life, and with the internalized father, the superego. Second, the use of this rivalry and the competitive struggle to ward off passive needs for security, acceptance, and unconscious longing for masochistic homosexual gratification. The constant belligerence disguises the desire to be loved. Submission serves as escape from the problem of rivalry. To put it in technical language: One wards off the positive Oedipus complex with the negative Oedipus complex, and vice versa; the respective attitudes can alternate in their role as defense against the corresponding opposite position. The defensive character is recognizable in the excessive degree of the reaction; it disturbs adaptation.

Work disturbances are psychodynamically not unlike the authority conflicts. "I do not want to work," frequently means, "Father demands that I work, but I do not want to work because complying with his demand would signify my submission to him." Such a passive role arouses too much anxiety. It means to be defeated and to succumb to a superior power.

For many to read and to study implies an injury to their self-esteem: "I have to read the book, really I could have written that book myself." Conscious and unconscious fantasies of grandeur often disturb the capacity to absorb knowledge. As soon as one recognizes these fantasies and is able to view them with some humor they no longer act as obstacles to work and study. In some cases they even stimulate the person's studies. Study requires our reading something not only once, but repeatedly. Many students have an ideal student in mind who can read a book once and remember forever every detail. In their discontent and anger about not being able to accomplish such a feat, they become unable to absorb the material read, give up in disgust, and turn to other pursuits. We also have to consider the superego and ego ideal problems in relation to work disturbances and authority conflicts. It should be emphasized once again that a symptom is connected with more than a single developmental phase. Work disturbances can also be based on an attitude of anal obstinacy. Revenge feelings for the frustrations experienced in the oral phase of development can lead to reluctance to give something to others.

We now shall review the phallic-narcissistic type. A popular representative of this type is the Don Juan figure of operatic fame. The man with a phallic-narcissistic character acts out his neurosis in his sexual life. The patients of this category are plagued by unconscious castration fears; they ward them off by a long series of sexual experiences which are meant to convince them of their unimpaired sexual power. These adventures are also to provide gratification of their drives with passive aims. The men identify with their female companions; here too the negative Oedipus complex is warded off with the help of the positive Oedipus complex.

The he-man has to be exceedingly masculine because he fears his own feminine traits.

The phallic-narcissistic attitude is often displaced to other areas than the sexual. Successes in these areas are then perceived as signs of virility. Gratification of passive needs is obtained by way of the admiration which these successful men receive from the environment. I refer to such characters as the Don Juan of success. The difference between the neurotic need to perform and the healthy desire to work is that the latter contains a genuine interest in and enjoyment of the work as such. Neurotic passion to accomplish great things merely uses work as the arena in which ambition and lust for fame strive for fulfillment. It is self-evident that there are many intermediate stages between normal joy in work and pathological addiction to performance. Between health and neurosis nature makes no sudden leaps. It is perfectly healthy to be pleased at a success; the distinction between normal and neurotic rests here as in many other instances on quantitative factors.

The sexual Don Juan is driven from woman to woman, the warded-off desire is not fully satisfied, and each woman is a disappointment to him. The hidden castration fears cause secret disdain and fear of the woman. The infatuation temporarily wards off the hidden feelings, but as soon as the woman has been won the disappointment rapidly follows. The Don Juan type is the male counterpart of the woman who tends towards neurotic faithlessness on the basis of her penis envy. Investigation of the psychopathology of both types reveals interesting parallels. A phallic-narcissistic man has sexual desires and believes he is in love, but cannot establish a lasting relationship. The same obtains for the woman with a phallic hysteria. The phallic-narcissistic man does not accept his sexual role. He identifies with his female partner, and would actually like to play the woman's role. Reacting against this, he has to play the role of a particularly virile man. The woman with phallic hysteria fails to accept her feminine role, she wants to be a man; she uses sexual relationships for the purpose of obtaining a penis. This effort in fantasy is as much in vain as the attempts of the neurotic man to gratify his feminine wishes. The pathology of both originates in the castration complex, in the castration fears of the man and the penis envy of the woman. We cannot examine all the parallels in detail. However, it should be pointed out that the domineering female type is the counterpart of the passive male. One could describe the domineering woman as phallic-narcissistic; she is, after all, pseudo masculine; she uses her intellect as a masculine attribute and is very proud of it. The man who cannot accept his own sexual role does not acquire the feminine traits of a normal woman. He displays traits corresponding to those of a neurotic woman. Some men have much in common with the castrating woman: their wooing for favors and love, their ostentation, their infidelity and their triumph in rejecting the partner.

One of the complications of the little boy's forsaking the competitive struggle and submitting to the father in the hope of gaining his love is the ensuing masochism.

The concept of masochism has many meanings. We refer to someone as masochistic whose severe conscience imposes punishment and suffering on him. For instance a young man spoils an evening with his girl friend by starting a quarrel over some trivial matter. It appears that he has to ruin everything he enjoys or anticipates enjoyment from. This self-punishment may be the result of rage directed at himself—one has to destroy oneself or a part of oneself, or at least prevent contentment and happiness. It is proper to regard the need for punishment as a disturbance of the intrapsychic relationship between ego and superego. The punishment is imposed by the superego, the ego submits to it to be reaccepted in love, in the same way in which the parent, having punished the child, forgives him and turns to him with love. They are all the more affectionate if the punishment turns out to be harsher than they had intended it to be. The intrapsychic relationships were originally the relationships of the child with his real or imaginary parents. When the ego accepts the imposition of a punishment so severe that the person's whole life becomes one continuous exercise of penitence we refer to moral masochism. The original "father beats me," which contained a mixture of sensual pleasure and defense against castration fears, becomes transformed into the impression that the person is a victim of repetitive blows of fate. The primary sexual problem is no longer accessible to conscious experience.

Sexual masochism is a perversion, i.e., sexual pleasure can be experienced only on condition that suffering and humiliation are intimately connected with it. Sexual masochism has different determinants. That pleasure can be experienced only in connection with pain and humiliation, can be the result of a fusion of forbidden pleasure and the penance for this pleasure. In the masochistic fantasies it is for the most part the buttocks that are being beaten. A comforting thought is hidden in this fantasy: "I am being punished but my genitals are safe from harm." It is remarkable that the fantasy of the masochistic man often conjures up the image of a masculine woman, equipped with riding crop, and dressed like the members of a motorcycle gang. The derivation of homosexuality from the negative Oedipus complex is clearly discernible. The fantasy "a woman beats me" conceals the wish to be beaten by a man or a phallic woman. This fantasy is a disguised elaboration of the wish to be loved by a man. The passive submission is a faulty resolution of the Oedipus complex.

Sometimes masochism has a different meaning. To be punished and to be beaten may be the only way in which a child receives attention. The child, fearful that his parents will abandon him, prefers punishment to loneliness; the pain of loneliness is so much worse than the pain of being beaten, that by comparison with the former the latter may acquire a pleasurable quality. This motivation is valid for sexual as well as moral masochism.

There is a close relationship between these two seemingly different phenomena. At first glance there is little in common between a student who fails his examination through ineptness and the young man who enjoys being whipped. Closer examination reveals a significant kinship between them. The inept student provokes misfortune and failure in order to be relieved of guilt feelings, and the redeeming of the guilt originally may have had a pleasurable character. Misfortune is often being perpetuated in order to hold on to this hidden, repressed pleasurable component. Nevertheless it would be a bad mistake to accuse a patient of wishing misfortune on himself.

Freud pointed out that man pursued by fate retains a hidden relationship to the impersonal punishing father. The pleasurable aspect of the masochistic attitude varies greatly; it is most pronounced in sexual masochism, and is lacking in moral masochism. A passive-feminine attitude conceals jealousy, masochism conceals sadistic fantasies.

We have described a series of neurotic patterns and types, all connected with the negative Oedipus complex. In conclusion one more general observation: Insight into the complicated interplay of forces between instinctual impulse and defense is a precondition for the comprehension of neurotic manifestations. Once the insight is obtained one can recognize the value of descriptive differentiation. There are significant clinical distinctions between the inhibited neurotic person, the phallic-narcissistic Don Juan figure and the passive homosexual man. Closer investigation reveals that the restrictions of the inhibited neurotic have the purpose of suppressing a Don Juan fantasy, and that this fantasy is used for the defense against passive homosexuality; the latter in turn is the result of a faulty resolution of the Oedipus complex. It is therefore very important to begin with a description of the case, without theoretical preconceptions. Then the described material should be fitted into the appropriate category, and then the psychic mechanisms should be further studied. Somatic and situational factors which may codetermine the manifestations of the neurosis, the perversion or psychopathy, should not be neglected.

Understanding the relationship between impulse and defense is indispensable for understanding the neurotic patient. The shyness of the yielding, inhibited and blushing girl may be the result of warded-off passion, her sexual longing may be a defense against penis envy, the penis envy itself may be a reaction to the disappointments in the oedipal relationship to her father.

The Oedipus complex is the nuclear complex of the neurosis; this formulation of Freud has not been invalidated. The defense changes with the person's development; as in geological formations, layer upon layer is superimposed on each other in the course of time. Unlike the sediments in geological processes, however, a defensive technique of earlier times can be used to ward off problems of a later age. A woman can again become infantile and dependent in order to avoid adult sexuality. Attitudes stemming from the earliest phase of development, the oral phase, may appear on the contemporary surface of psychic events. Regression sometimes confuses the observer, he feels confronted by a chaotic picture. Careful attention to the relationships between defense and instinctual impulse helps us to recognize that the chaotic condition is not real. To clarify what is meant by the foregoing observations, I should like to offer one last example: A young man is shy, modest and withdrawn. He is ashamed of his masochistic fantasies, in which he sees himself beaten by boys, and in which he seeks protection from a maternal figure. The regression is evident here. The masochistic submission and the wish to be sheltered is an attempt to escape the anxieties engendered by his heterosexual wishes. Passive attitudes are used to avoid the dangers of a masculine position. A developmentally earlier attitude serves to ward off problems of a later stage.

ON THE COURSE OF THE DISORDER

Some remarks about the course of the hysterical neuroses should be added here. Prediction in this matter is difficult. The prognosis is determined by the degree of the neurotic conflict, by dispositional factors and by the patient's reality situation. The course is often very capricious.

Conversion symptoms can take a malignant course, and result in invalidism, necessitating hospitalization. Anxiety hysterias can remain limited for years to one insignificant symptom, but they can also spread out and result in an incapacitating restriction of the patient's mobility. The choice of marriage partner often determines whether a relative equilibrium and a more or less adequate adaptation can be established. The whole family can be drawn into the neurosis. The course of the disease is then largely determined by the ensuing situation.

Female patients of the revenge type display conspicuous variations of the hysterical manifestations. When no object for infatuation is available the patient suffers from a nostalgic depression. When she has won a lover, there is a short period of lively, even exuberant reaction, and this is followed by doubts, and, in some cases, by conversion symptoms. At times the triumphant reaction associated with the rejection of the lover reaches almost maniacal proportions. The music and the lyrics of the final great aria in Richard Strauss' opera *Salome* express magnificently the turmoil of these emotions. Some women of this type must pay dearly for their revenge;

they forever long for the rejected man and react with a neurotic depression with or without conversion symptoms. Some sado-masochistic characters alternate between the sadistic and masochistic positions.

In my opinion many menopausal depressions are in reality decompensated hysterical neuroses. They occur at the time when the children leave home. The children no longer can be perceived as extensions of the patient, and her labile psychic equilibrium is disrupted.

The male counterpart of the revenge type, the phallic-narcissistic patient, acts out his neurosis inconspicuously. The adaptation succeeds at the price of suffering which the triangular situations inflict on the patient and his women. In such situations one sees periods of infatuation and depression in rapid alternation.

Upon reflecting that there are inumerable transitional phenomena between psychic health and severe neurosis, and that the healthy aspects of the personality also influence the course of the affliction, we have to admit that there is not much we can definitely say about it. Life brings about many surprises for us and for the patient. Situational factors can bring about changes which we sometimes regard as nothing less than miraculous.

6

NEURASTHENIA
AND THE SENSITIVE PERSONALITY

IN ADDITION to the already-described character neuroses two other categories occurring in clinical practice are to be mentioned, neurasthenia and the sensitive personality. I am acquainted with many psychiatrists who do not wish to forego further differentiation of the neurotic personalities, and I too believe it is justified to call attention to these character formations.

Some leading psychiatrists have investigated these clinical categories and have proposed some unifying classification guidelines: Kretschmer developed his characterology, in which he included the sensitive personality type. Carp (1947) investigated the neurotic and psychopathic types with the help of anthropological and psychoanalytical data. He raised the level of clinical differentiation above that of an unsystematic description. He treats the neurasthenic personality as part of the neuroses, the sensitive personality as an aspect of the psychopathic disorders. At all times he endeavors to combine clinical and psychoanalytic conceptualizations. Du Boeuff favored the tripartite differentiation into hysterical, neurasthenic and sensitive character forms. He described all of these conditions as deficient operations of various modes of being.

In investigating the different characterological entities we must direct our attention to three aspects of the person: his general endowment, his temperament, and the manner in which he deals with his instinctual impulses. The last item involves matters like the relative roles of sublimation, of action and of defense. The most promising approach is one of a dynamically and genetically oriented characterology. The formation of the character represents a form of adaptation. We shall best understand it by investigating the significance of the person's attitudes and actions in regard to his environment and to his own instinctual impulses. We must also learn how these different aspects of his behavior developed. We can recognize the healthy person by his ability to strive for optimal adaptation. The neurotic and psychopathic character features are rigid and poorly adapted.

We cannot give a comprehensive account of all attempts to organize the neurotic character manifestations into systematic orders. Jung and Van der Hoop have proposed a classification; Klages suggested a characterology which at one time was applied in psychiatry, and many others could be named. I shall limit myself to a description of those categories which appear to me most serviceable in the psychiatrist's daily practice, and shall approach the subject from the dynamic and genetic points of view.

We shall take the neurasthenic conditions first. Chryzanowski (1959) writes in the *American Handbook of Psychiatry:*

> We are dealing here with time-honored concepts which have a most undynamic quality. From an operational viewpoint, neurasthenia and hypochondriasis are awkward, antiquated pieces of furniture, not much good for anything. Nevertheless, both terms have gained a powerful foothold in psychiatric terminology. For the time being, they seem to be here to stay; rather than complain unduly or coin new names, we may as well look

into the nature and the implications of the old-fashioned terms as they appear in sundry clinical phenomena [p. 258].

The symptoms of the neurasthenic neuroses are vague complaints of fatigue, headache, backache, stomach distress and others. They are often accented by a hypochondriacal overtone. Accordingly, in the *American Handbook,* neurasthenia and hypochondriasis are treated together. The patients also complain of a feeling of anxious tension, accompanied by cardiac palpitation, perspiration and oppression. These last-mentioned symptoms can be so severe that the physician is inclined to think of a thyrotoxic illness. Many thyroid glands of neurasthenic patients have been removed by unsuspecting surgeons. The neurasthenic anxiety frequently takes the form of fear of failure. Without doubt, the less serious exogenic reactions of hyperaesthesia are frequently and mistakenly regarded as a part of the neurasthenic syndrome. The complaints of neurasthenic patients do indeed show much similarity with the symptoms of patients whose so-called irritable weakness is caused by exogenic factors. Both groups are hypersensitive, intolerant of excitation and of psychic stress; they complain of fatigue, difficulty in concentration, and various symptoms involving the sympathetic nervous system. Following Stern, who coined the term, these conditions can be described as "mental-physical-neutral." The fatigue is simultaneously a mental and physical experience, as are restlessness and sleep disturbances. The investigator will find accentuated reflexes, demographism, a labile pulse rate and general tension. The latter often represents a reaction to the examination. The patients appear exhausted and pale. Their mental symptoms are feelings of insufficiency, they complain of not being able to accomplish anything worthwhile: "They could do much more if only they were not so weak and flabby." We shall see later that the feelings of insufficiency are the cause not the effect of the weakness and lassitude. These feelings influence the interpersonal relationships: neurasthenic patients often believe that the environment shares their own evaluation of themselves as insufficient. Such patients are often known to be conscientious and dutiful people. These traits are sometimes exaggerated to a degree which makes one think of a compulsive character. It is quite possible that neurasthenia is, in the dynamic and genetic sense, related to compulsive neurosis. However, as a rule the emotional rigidity is not as prominent in the neurasthenics as in typical compulsive characters. Among the patients' ego-syntonic feelings those of insufficiency and the conviction that they are considered a failure by others are much in the foreground. As far as their sexuality is concerned it has a hypochondriacal aspect; the patients ascribe their fatigue to their sexual activities. A typical example is that of an official who has intercourse with his wife only on Saturday nights, on the eve of national holidays and during vacations. When he occasionally broke his own rule he feared that he would be fatigued, and make mistakes in his work the next day. (Indeed, he had a peculiar feeling in his body, his back ached and his head felt heavy.)

Those doctors who pay attention only to bodily complaints and hold that psychogenic manifestations are unreal relate differently to neurasthenical and to hysterical complaints. The hysterical patients are designated as pretenders, the neurasthenics as grouches, and their complaints as whining or belly-aching. Disparaging judgments, however, sometimes contain phenomenological descriptions which are usable once they are translated into somewhat less disapproving terms. The doctors respond to the observation that some hysterical patients display a certain animation, and are oriented towards the listener, while the neurasthenic patients appear spiritless and disinterested. The neurasthenic patient is not given to pseudo emotionality like the hysterical patients, who never cease to experiment with interpersonal relationships in their quest for attention. Furthermore it must be pointed out that neurasthenic patients too are inclined towards hypersensitive emotional reactions. It appears that they never have enough mental energy, and that even minor disturbances of cerebral function result in decompensation. Small wonder that these patients have again and again been thought of as genetically predisposed towards their problems. Indeed, one encounters among them fairly often a definite constitutional type, the asthenic body type described by Stiller. The same complaints are often voiced by patients of the leptosome type, but it is very difficult to image a pyknic neurasthenic. The parasympathetic lability and the symptoms involving both psyche and body can be viewed as a consequence of the neurosis. One can probably not say the same of the constitutional features. It is unlikely to be merely coincidental that patients in the initial phase of psychoses and patients recovering from an infectious disease have approximately the same complaints as the neurasthenic patients. One receives the impression in all three instances that the energy required for adaptation is insufficient.

Some psychiatrists use the concept of psychasthenia; the psychasthenic person is characterized by precision, compulsiveness, and scrupulousness. Psychasthenia seems to be a transitional condition between neurasthenia and the conpulsive character neuroses. The symptomatology of psychasthenic patients includes ties, phobias, and obsessive-compulsive manifestations. The patients also have a tendency to derealization and depersonalization. There occurs a loss of contact with reality caused by a general diminution of the available psychic energy, and there is a lowering of the general mental performance level. The question may be raised: Are these conditions neurotic manifestations or expressions of a constitutional defect? In my opinion the answer is that we see in these conditions an interaction of both factors at work.

Van Dantzig and Waage (1962) observed the preponderance of a feeling of helplessness and apathy that accompanies neurasthenic reactions. They see these feelings as a sign of decompensation. Fatigue, feebleness, and apathy can be designated as the basic symptoms of the neurasthenic character.

Many symptoms and difficulties in human relationships which are reminiscent of hysteria and are to be found in neurasthenic patients occur also in people of the sensitive character type described by Kretschmer (1927). It is often said that French psychiatry was mainly interested in hallucinations whereas delusions aroused the interest of German psychiatry. The delineation of the sensitive character type is indeed closely related to the problem of delusional manifestations. Kretschmer described genuine delusions in nonschizophrenic patients. He ascribes this delusion to a specific interaction between the patient's character and his environment. Of particular importance is the undermining of self-esteem which occurs in these patients prior to the appearance of the delusion. The problem of the sensitive character is based on related circumstances. The patients are particularly sensitive to all impressions and stimuli that impinge on them. They are not, however, capable of adequately discharging the emotional tension. They experience the exaggerated sensitivity sometimes as ego-syntonic, as justified, and at other times as inappropriate, in which case they make efforts to overcome it. One cannot say that they react only to injuries to their own self-esteem. They respond very strongly to the unhappiness and pain of others, but are unable to express their own feelings freely. They find life hard. Kretschmer mentioned the strict conscience of the sensitive character types. Indeed they are troubled by guilt feelings and scruples. Among their complaints we encounter fleeting paranoid manifestations. They have a vague feeling that others are against them. They sometimes become depressed in reaction to mild offences. The paranoid and depressive reactions often are disguised by headaches, sleep disturbances, fatigue, disturbances of consciousness and hypochondriacal symptoms. There is a strong resemblance to the neurasthenic symptomatology. However, the complaints appear to express a feeling of loneliness and insecurity rather than an inability to realize ideals. In their interactions with others the people with features of the sensitive character show a superficial similarity with hysterical patients. They fear loss of love.

We must not neglect to mention the positive aspects of the neurasthenic and sensitive personalities. Neurasthenic people often have a pronounced sense of duty; the sensitive person is characterized by what could be called his "emotional gifts," i.e., his awareness of and responsiveness to emotions of others.

Differentiation of the various character types is not easy; unfortunately the physician's own unconscious emotions interfere in his making an objective diagnosis. The sensitive character is sometimes seen as a hysterical personality because the patient's symptoms arouse anxiety in the doctor. Once again it should be emphasized that accurate psychoanalytic knowledge about the operation of the ego functions, the defenses, the superego and their attitude to the drives is necessary for the understanding of neurasthenia in genetic and dynamic terms.

It is possible that neurasthenic patients are afflicted with a constitutional "weakness" of the capacity to establish emotional relationships, but to ascribe the patient's failures to this one factor would be a one-sided and narrow view. Unresolved problems of the infantile instinctual life are at least as important as the constitutional factor. In many patients the inhibition has pre-oedipal roots. The fear of being rejected is so intense that no relationships at all are formed. This fear is also to be found in neuroses which are reminiscent of neurasthenic conditions. Other inhibitions are related to the oedipal problems. Latent homosexuality causes fear of intimacy with persons of the same sex. Feelings of guilt, hypochondriacal and paranoid elaborations of the oedipal problem interfere with love relationships. The inhibition of genital sexuality, however, is not a predominant problem in these characters.

Carp (1947) recognized an essential characteristic of the neurasthenic person in the tension between his ego ideal and his realistic ability:

> The neurasthenic forms of being have their roots in the too tautly stretched desire to live a life corresponding to their capacity for subjective experience, but not to their realistic capacity for performance. This situation contains a permanent conflict, which is constantly rekindled by doubts about the value of their experience [p. 292].

The neurasthenic patient is exhorted by his ego ideal to commit himself to high ideals and to sacrifice himself for his fellow human beings, but this is precisely what his unresolved instinctual conflicts prevent him from doing. It becomes clear why the hysterical neuroses are more common among women, and the neurasthenic conditions more common among men. It is easy to induce the girl to form an ego ideal which approves of love. This does not imply that her education will help her to realize that ideal. Unfortunately the wish to rear the girl to become a good mother is all too often accompanied by a rigid suppression of her sexuality. The boys are for the most part reared to be successful or idealistic men, not good lovers. At the same time the energy sources necessary to serve an ideal or achieve a significant goal are blocked. In my opinion the inhibition of aggression is also of great significance in these character formations. Here too we find discrepancy between the demands of the superego and of the ego ideal. The ego ideal prescribes a conduct impossible to realize, owing to the defenses which are kept active by the influence of the superego.

These considerations help us to understand more about the fatigue, the difficulty in concentration and the fear of failure. We know that incomplete or faulty integration of the aggressive instinctual impulses seriously interferes with a man's capacity to work. The aggressive drive has been disturbed in its development, the infantile forms of the drive are being warded off, and the ego functions cannot support adult creative activity. In addition the defenses use up a significant portion of the person's psychic energy. Disturbances of ego consciousness and manifestations of derealization are also caused by the inhibition of aggression. It is my impression that the neurasthenic patients also employ defenses characteristic of the compulsive neurotics, for instance, the warding off of affect and the isolation of content from the affect. The compulsive character is more rigid than the neurasthenic character and there are probably some typical differences in their ego ideals. The neurasthenic patient's ego ideal is also quite different from the ego ideal of the hysterical patient. He employs different defense techniques which make the establishment of human relationships particularly difficult for him. His secret fantasies of grandeur result in his constantly being disappointed in himself; he seeks to soothe the resulting injury to his self-esteem by unconsciously thinking of himself in still more exalted terms, and this of necessity results in further injured feelings.

The inhibition of aggression is no less prominent in the sensitive character. They express their hurt feelings no more than the neurasthenic characters. But while the neurasthenic patient energetically wards off his passive needs, the sensitive personality type is able to utilize them for his adaptation. The infantile passive strivings, expressed in the wishes to be accepted, sheltered, and cared for, lend themselves to this purpose for the following reasons: The patient's self-esteem is greater when he succeeds in warding off anger, jealousy and other aggressive manifestations with the help of the dependent attitude. These people avoid all competition, and manage with the help of their environment to achieve a relative degree of adaptation. Passivity prevails in their love life as well, for them love means to be sustained by expressions of love that others direct to them. When they receive love they are also able to love. Their sexual and erotic behavior is reminiscent of the attitudes between mother and child. I have termed this attitude a "passive adaptation." We shall return to the subject in the chapter on depressions.

It is evident that the environment cannot meet the expectations and demands of the sensitive character types. They feel that they do not get recognition for their work and feel misunderstood in their marriages. Decompensation readily occurs, and depressive, paranoid or neurasthenic reactions follow in its wake.

Of course not everyone using this passive form of adaptation is a sensitive personality. Many people who are not very active in their love life, lack courage, and are not very alert, do not show the moral preoccupation of the sensitive personality, nor do they inhibit their aggressiveness but respond to provocation in a vigorous manner. Du Boeuff designated all those who depend on others for support of their self-esteem, and who adapt to the environment like a water lily to the water as "relationists." This group encompasses all those who prefer a passive adaptation. It includes the sensitive personalities.

Finally, I hope that I have succeeded in showing that many character variations within the hysterical neuroses originate not only in the phallic phase, but also have pre-oedipal vicissitudes.

7

───────◆◆◆◆◆◆◆───────

OBSESSIVE-COMPULSIVE
NEUROSIS

WE HAVE briefly mentioned the compulsive manifestations when we discussed their function as defense against anxiety. We speak of compulsive phenomena when the ego in vain resists their appearance, and feels helpless in its struggle against them. This leads us to philosophical problems. There are not many symptoms of mental illness equally concerned with the dialectics of free will and its absence in man's existence. To avoid keeping our observations on a too abstract plane let us review a few examples:

A patient can neither begin nor finish his day without giving in to his washing compulsion. He fears that he might have touched things that are "contaminated" with menstrual blood. His apprehensions make it impossible for him to walk through the main shopping area of his city, or to visit a museum.

Another patient, a woman from a puritanical, religious background, is offended by a compulsive image which enters her mind while she is at church. The minister's wife looks reverently at her husband who moves his bowels into a chamberpot in the corner. The wife holds the pot so that she catches his feces in it.

Compulsive images are often in sharp contrast to the situation in which they inflict themselves on the patient, as is abundantly demonstrated by the preceding example. In the first example the compulsion is related to the realm of genital sexuality, in the second the subject is undisguisedly anal. The next example illustrates the connection between compulsion and doubt. A schoolgirl has to repeat rapidly after each statement the following words: "I believe, I believe, I believe . . ." Asked why she is saying this she replies: "It is possible that I have said something that is not true, that I have lied. I never know it for certain, and therefore I must say, 'I believe,' because when I say that, I cannot lie."

Some compulsive manifestations result in the avoidance of specific situations. A student fears that he will stand up in class during an admired professor's lecture and loudly call out a name cleverly composed of a vernacular expression for "homosexual" and the professor's specialty. He dares not attend the professor's class. The reader acquainted with depth psychology will readily recognize that this student wards off fantasies of a homosexual seduction. In this case the compulsive symptom is connected with a phobia.

Finally, an example of obsessive thoughts permeated with doubts, which Adolf Meyer termed "obsessive rumination." The patient is compelled to think of metaphysical problems, which are reminiscent of the queries of children, like, "Why is the earth round and not rectangular? Why does the sea reach only to the beach?"

Compulsive inhibition has to be mentioned since it plays a large role in work disturbances. A patient intends to study a scientific paper, but as she sits down to her reading she is overwhelmed by the thought that first she has to answer a friend's letter, or she has to bring order to her desk, or to do some laundry. Very common is the compulsion to interpose activities such as housecleaning, tidying, etc., before one starts on any task. It is one of the commonest work disturbances. The reader will have no difficulty in recognizing that the obsessive phenomenon is super-imposed on the ego's general experience, and that the ego is unable to resist this process. This helplessness is often so painful that a reaction of utter despair and anguish sets in and severely incapacitates the patient.

We can now proceed to discuss the peculiar dialectic personality structure of human beings which makes such obsessive phenomena possible. This is not the same as discussing the origin of the obsessions. The possibility of obsessive and compulsive manifestations rests on the philosophical fact that man who experiences himself as master of his mind and body and as free agent in the interaction with his environment, is nevertheless motivated by factors which are rooted in his past. At the height of his experience of inner freedom he will maintain: "I have no alternative choice," and will repeat Luther's "Here I stand, I cannot do otherwise." To illustrate this: If a young man, who is deeply in love with a girl were to be asked whether he is being forced to become engaged to her, he would look astonished at the question. "Being forced? Certainly not! I have never undertaken anything in my life which was more of a free decision than this engagement." Yet, the young man arrived at the choice of his fiancée on the basis of conscious and unconscious factors which determine his motives. His action is both free and determined by motives of which he is unaware. It is an action of his free will, yet he could not act differently without becoming untrue to himself.

By free we mean neither the freedom to desire everything nor the power to enforce our desires, but the ability to evaluate our motives with discrimination, the willingness to affirm the forces which determine our existence, and the capacity to act appropriately on a decision, when the circumstances permit it. We live in inner harmony when our freedom and our awareness of what determines us coincide. The ego, the center of our personality, can claim as its own what belongs to the self—our conscience, our instinctual life, our past. In resisting the forces impinging on us as well as in cooperating with these forces the ego experiences itself as a free agent. Disturbances in the ego result in various forms of impairment of the ego's freedom of choice and action. The compulsive symptoms belong in this category. The compulsion is a disturbance in the experience of one's own activity. Kronfeld (1930) states: "In so far as the ego's central activity is involved in ideas, judgments, fears, apprehensions, expectations and the assumption of definite positions, all these areas are subject to anomalies in the experience of activity."

There are many forms of disturbances of this experience. To understand them we approach the matter from psychoanalytic perspective and use the term *ego* in the psychoanalytic sense. The ego can admit a drive derivative into consciousness, it can approve of it and turn it into an action. If met by no resistance from conscience and from the environment we expect this action to be accompanied by a pleasurable discharge. The affects associated with it are of a positive nature, reaching from the experience of mild pleasure to ecstatic gratitude. The positive coloring of the affective experience is to a large degree the result of the experience that one's action is in harmony with oneself and with the world.

However, when an intense impulse has to be controlled because it is not in harmony with conscience and the environment, the ego has at its disposal different techniques. The best is mastery. Mastery implies an inner conflict. The experience of inner freedom is not changed thereby, but the feeling tone moves towards the negative pole of the scale. In this conflict the person is honest towards himself. That it is necessary to master not only instinctual impulses but the conscience is often disregarded or forgotten. For example: A strictly-reared man, during whose childhood and youth visits to the cinema were forbidden to him, accompanies his wife to view a film, yet he feels restless and vaguely discontented while they are in the movie theater. Still, he is able to fulfill his wife's wish; his ego, supported by the reasonable part of his conscience, can dismiss the influence of the archaic prohibitive part of his conscience. Not only instinctual impulses but also conscience demands can be mastered given a strong ego that can bear conflict.

When conflicts have their roots in childhood they cause so much anxiety that defense mechanisms have to be utilized by the ego. One of the most important defenses is repression. When a strong instinctual impulse strives to break through to consciousness diffuse anxiety appears. When a specific situation represents a particular temptation for the drive this situation is avoided. In that case we refer to a phobic defense. Other defenses are called into action when repression alone is insufficient, for example reversal into the opposite. The lecherous person turns into a fanatical defender of decency.

When the ego is overrun by drive derivatives which assert themselves against its will, and it is not cognizant of their source, the ego feels overwhelmed. A particularly intense negative affect accompanies this circumstance. The breakdown of the ego's subjective experience of freedom is perceived as very painful. The intensive yet vain struggle of the ego against a drive derivative which is breaking through the consciousness is experienced as compulsion. This relationship between ego and instinctual impulse is distinguished from a normal conflict between drive and conscience. For example, in the conflict experienced by a man about to engage in a sexual affair disapproved by his conscience there is no disturbance of the feeling that one is master of one's activity. Perhaps the man is being seduced, but he does not feel helplessly driven by an immutable compulsion. In fact, he takes the side of the drive in the conflict; were he not to take its side, all pleasure in the affair would escape him. Man experiences himself as determining his thoughts and actions in masturbation conflicts also. After the drive is satisfied guilt feelings may set in, but a person who gives in to a compulsion experiences no pleasure whatever, and afterward he is desperate and unhappy rather than guilty. The impulse involved in a compulsive symptom is more ego-alien than is a conflict between drive and a more or less masterful ego. But though it is ego-alien, it is not alien to the self. The compulsive neurotic never accuses others of influencing his thoughts, or of producing ideas in his mind. It is characteristic of the tormenting nature of the compulsive manifestations that they are perceived as belonging to one's personality. When the compelling idea is experienced as coming from outside, and the ego feels influenced by others in its thoughts and actions, we speak no longer of a compulsive symptom but of paranoid delusions.

A condition for the appearance of compulsive symptoms now becomes clear. The compulsion presupposes an ego which reacts to primitive instinctual impulses with a vehement rejection and at the same time is under threat of a very severe conscience. The question may be raised how does it happen that an ego gets into such a bitter feud with its conscience and with the drive? The ego landed in its predicament because of a disturbance in the development of the infantile instinctual life. An example would be the case of the patient with the compulsive avoidance of menstrual blood that I mentioned before. Here the infantile sexual impulses are not very concealed though they appear in warded-off form.

Many investigators have noted that obsessive-compulsive patients are preoccupied with the subject of soiling and contamination. In one of the examples above the infantile curiosity about the excretory function came to the fore quite openly. The compulsive neurotic is not troubled by impulses which have their origin in adult instinctual life. While the hysterical patient wards off the oedipal strivings by means of repression and reversal into the opposite, the obsessional patient utilizes another, more complicated defense mechanism, i.e., regression. Freud (1918) pointed out two meanings of regression: (1) retreat from a danger; and (2) return to a previous stage of development. The obsessional patient seeks refuge in the gratifications of the anal phase of development in order to escape the unbearable feelings of guilt and the anxiety generated by the oedipal problems. But he does not find the refuge he seeks; he cannot give in to the anal impulses; instead they are warded off by means of reversal and other defense mechanisms. In this struggle against the drive the conscience has become excessively severe. It is very punitive and behaves much more harshly than the parents ever did. The ego sides neither with the id impulses rooted in the infantile instinctual drives, nor with the harsh demands of its conscience, rather, it has become a helpless victim of both forces. The compulsive and obsessional symptoms contain both the impulses of the id and the punishment of the superego. The compulsion to call the professor a homosexual is the result of a breakthrough of an id impulse.

I should like to emphasize once more the typical aspects of the obsessive compulsive symptomatology.

The person does not experience the obsessive manifestations as belonging to his ego; the ego does not approve of them, it rejects them. The attempts at their suppression are experienced as in vain, and are accompanied by a feeling of helplessness. Whether the suppression is successful or not, the ego feels helpless in either case. The ego struggles with the compulsion, and is acutely aware of the danger of losing its struggle. It experiences itself as helpless, dominated, unfree, and obsessed. It experiences its resistance against the compulsive symptoms as an action of its free will in the struggle against the compulsion [trans. from Kronfeld, 1930, p. 217].

The clinical usage applies the expression "obsessive" to actions which had better be termed "driven," as for instance, in the case of a man who is driven to flirt with every woman he meets, or the woman who is constantly driven to engage in arguments.

When the central activity of the ego is disturbed every psychic phenomenon can acquire an obsessive quality. We shall examine the obsessive involvement of the functions of perception, imagination and thought, of impulses and actions, and also review briefly the relationship between obsession and affect.

Are there compulsive perceptions? An example of one is the compulsion to check repeatedly whether the door is truly locked, the gas jet securely turned off, the light switched off in every room, etc. The compulsion is attached to doubts which are rooted in conflicts of ambivalence. Should I or shouldn't I harm the people in the house (by admitting the burglar, by turning on the gas, etc.). In such instances obsession and doubt are closely interwoven. Mental images are often imbued with obsessional qualities. The obsession in that case is an unconscious fantasy which breaks through into consciousness against the resistance of the ego. The fantasies are experienced pictorially as mental images. The obsessive phenomenon is often described beginning with the words: "I imagine that . . ."

Since the cooperation of the ego is necessary for the production of mental images, and the ego invariably refuses its cooperation, the images of the obsessional neurotic, unlike the elaborate fantasies of the hysteric, have a fleeting character, and disappear from awareness as fast as they appear. Sometimes the compulsion produces no more than a sudden brief impression. A melody can pursue one, or a single line from a poem can suddenly appear in one's mind with obsessive insistence. There is a gradual transition between mental imagery and thought. In thought word symbols replace the visual or acoustic content.

There are many kinds of obsessive thoughts. Often divergent and incompatible ideas are brought together in one obsessive thought. The churchgoer has to think of an obscene subject or he is unable to prevent the emergence of a ridiculous idea in his mind while he takes part in some solemn social function. The process of thought itself can be obsessive. The endless pondering of a question, the painstaking review of a subject from all possible angles, are examples of obsessive thought. The topics of such obsessive thought processes are commonly the meaning of life, the finite and infinite, free will and determinism, predestination and personal responsibility and other similar subjects. Fenichel (1945) observed in regard to obsessive thought that this symptom is based on the attempt to avoid unpleasant emotions through retreat from the world of feeling into the world of intellectual concepts and words. He also describes an excellent example of obsessive thinking:

> A patient, looking at a door, was compelled to spend much time brooding about the problem: What is the main thing, the empty space, filled out by the door, or the substantial door, filling out the empty space? This 'philosophical' problem covered the doubt: What is the main thing in sexuality, woman or man? [p. 297].

Doubt can also be conceived as a manifestation of obsessive thinking: "Did I post the letter or not? Did I send the letter to my girl in which I referred to our sexual intercourse to her, or to my future mother-in-law? Did I send the letter intended for my mother-in-law to my fiancée?" etc.

In some cases it is difficult to draw the line between an obsessional and delusional idea. For example: "I cannot dismiss the thought that I have a venereal disease, in spite of my certain knowledge that I cannot possibly have contracted one." Or: "I cannot help thinking that I have sinned against the Holy Ghost." "I know very well that I am not responsible for my father's death, but the thought that I am guilty of it keeps entering my mind." Similar reports are commonly heard in practice. One could assume that people with such hypochondriacal and morbid preoccupations are in fact suffering from a phobic condition, in which the morbid fears have assumed an obsessive character. However, I believe we must avoid the mistake which our obsessive neurotic patients make so readily, i.e., the mistake of substituting an "either-or" for an "as well as." A hypochondriacal manifestation has many aspects; it may contain delusional imagery, phobic patterns, and also obsessive imagery. Delusional images are often subject to doubt, expressed in formulations like the following: "It disturbs me greatly that . . . I fear greatly that . . ." etc. Genuine delusions are experienced differently. The ego is convinced of their truth. A patient suffering from a genuine delusion of jealousy does not say: "I cannot free myself from the idea that my wife has an affair with another man." He says: "I am certain that she is not faithful to me." Du Boeuff rightly pointed out that the patients find some relief in this certainty. Obsessive thinking includes also the counting obsession. Sometimes obsessive counting is a punishment imposed by the superego. At other times it is a derivative of hidden sexual thoughts, and sometimes both simultaneously. Kronfeld (1930) refers to compulsive impulses or compulsions when the obsessional manifestation is expressed in an action. A compulsive impulse was present in the case of the student who felt impelled to call his professor a homosexual. In many cases the compulsion is connected with magical thinking: "If I do not cross the street before the red light goes on mother will die." Many children and adults feel compelled to step on every third or fourth crack in the pavement, so that . . . and then there follows the respective wish or fear magically connected with the trivial action.

Can affects be compulsive? First of all it must be pointed out that the obsession is invariably accompanied by an unpleasant affect, which can reach desperate proportions. Kraepelin and Aschaffenburg have pointed out that the compulsion is a disturbance of affectivity. When the obsessive manifestation is a recognizable consequence of an instinctual impulse the person's self-esteem is offended: "How can I think a thing like that?" When the conscience imposes a compulsion the ego feels maltreated. The phobias have an odd relationship with compulsive phenomena. In their case one could speak of compulsive affect. Indeed Kronfeld (1930) labels the phobia a "compulsive apprehension." Does such an approach contribute to a clarification? The fears are irrational, but are they also obsessional? I prefer to say that phobia initiates and motivates compulsive actions. A classical example is the washing compulsion. The content of the corresponding phobia is the fear of contamination with bacteria, feces, seminal fluid, etc. In obedience to the exhortations of his superego, the patient must clean himself of the "bad" substances.

A few cautionary remarks in regard to the compulsive impulses which can initiate compulsive actions are in order. It is not uncommon that hysterical patients who threaten suicide are dismissed with the comment that those who talk about it do not commit suicide. There are so many exemptions to this rule that to let the matter rest at that would be to err grievously. Many a hysterical patient has taken his life. The same applies to the compulsive neurotic patient.

The nurse on the obstetrical ward who cannot see a knife without thinking, "I must cut the baby's throat," will as a rule do no such thing. However, such an action by a nurse is not absolutely impossible, it could happen. One must carefully weigh the risks in such a situation and not be lulled into a false security by the notion that "a compulsive neurotic never gives in to his compulsive impulses."

Rituals and ceremonials can also have an anxiety mitigating significance: "If I do not fulfill the prescribed ceremony disaster will befall me." Compulsive manifestations are in many ways reminiscent of the experiences and ceremonies characteristic of primitive religions. Certain actions are executed in order to placate the gods. This similarity is not accidental. The compulsive neurotic patient is ruled by a tyrannical, pitiless superego which punishes the ego and demands penance from it. The hypothesis that the gods represent projections of a part of the believers' personality takes its departure from these considerations.

In some cases the compulsion becomes evident only in the inhibition which is its result. This can be clearly seen in work disturbances. A student sits down at his desk to study, but first he must tidy his desk, finish a letter, kill an annoying fly, etc. Not infrequently, opposition to the person on whose behalf the work is to be done is expressed in this fashion. The internal revolt creates the compulsion: "I cannot do what I should do, I am compelled to do something else first."

We have surveyed the compulsive manifestations and examined the question of what kind of psychic phenomena can become subjects of compulsion. We followed up Kronfeld's idea, that in true obsessive-compulsive conditions the compulsion must be experienced as such. In that sense we have found that there are compulsive perceptions and imagery; obsessive ideas, thoughts, and obsessive thinking but no compulsive phobias. The content of an obsessive thought carries the obsessive quality. In obsessive thinking the thinking process itself is contaminated by the obsession. We have also heard of compulsive impulses and learned that every compulsion invariably is accompanied by an affective reaction. The compulsion is primarily a disturbance in the conative realm, but it also involves the emotional areas of a person's life. We shall now turn to the examination of the compulsive neurotic patient's ego functions, his instinctual life and his superego functions.

The obsessive-compulsive patient utilizes different defense mechanisms than the hysterical patient. While the latter employs repression and projection, and strengthens the repression with the help of reversal, the former uses the mechanisms of isolation, rationalization and undoing. These are the predominant but not the only defense mechanisms found in obsessive neuroses. The obsessive neurotic also projects, and uses displacement of affect., i.e., he directs to one person what is meant for another, and he turns hostility on himself. His use of these defense mechanisms is not as consistent or as specific as his employment of the first-named three mechanisms of isolation, rationalization and undoing.

The obsessive patient separates and keeps apart what in reality belongs together. We say he isolates. The sudden thrusting into consciousness of an image, as in the example of the woman who sees the minister and his wife occupied with anal activities is a consequence of isolation. For purposes of clarification let us compare this obsessive image with the experiences of a child in a period when he is curious about the excretory functions and products. Children at that stage readily employ "bad" words which evoke smiles and laughter from siblings and friends. They want to enter the bathroom when one or the other of their parents is there and generally show much interest in the excretory functions of their family and of others. "Does the minister have to go to the bathroom like us?" is a type of question raised by the child. The occurrence of such questions during the nursery age is a source of harmless amusement; as the child grows they lose their significance. This is not, however, the case with the obsessive neurotic person. It is true, he no longer knows anything about these childhood events and he does not remember the prohibitions which were imposed on his curiosity. All that is present is an isolated image that thrusts itself into his mind, and he knows nothing of its origin. Many similar examples could be added here. Isolation is not limited to the content of ideas; cognitive and emotional aspects of ideas are also subjects of isolation. To put it in less technical language, in isolation the affect is separated from the content of ideas and images. Unlike the hysterical patient whose amnesia for childhood events is absolute, the compulsive patient can sometimes report events from his early years, but he mentions only pale, isolated facts, detached from his emotional experience.

Another defense mechanism closely connected with this isolation of affect and content is rationalization. Actions motivated by emotions stemming from instinctual life are "reasonably" explained and provided with a precise rationale. I heard a patient "explain" his sexual relationships in the following "rational" way: "We engage in sex for hygienic reasons, you understand, sexual tensions, unless discharged, are unhealthy."

The obsessive patient uses thought processes in place of emotional arguments; he does so even in situations where an emotional approach would be more adequate. This type of thinking is, of course, deficient, since thought in the service of a creative adaptation is invariably accompanied by the corresponding emotions. Compulsive thinking is characterized by certain specific qualities. It is magical thinking. Viewed genetically, the compulsive neurotic's experience is determined by regression to and fixation on the anal phase of development. Regression has occurred because of his failure to resolve the Oedipus complex. Guilt feelings, castration fears, jealousy and death wishes have not been overcome and are repressed. This is also the period in which thinking begins to develop. The ego learns to make use of this newly acquired function in the service of its defensive activity. It is thought that rapid development of ego functions may favor a disposition towards compulsion neurosis. At any rate, obsessional patients are often found to be unusually intelligent.

Early thinking is not realistic but magical. Inner world and external reality are not as yet sharply differentiated. Symbol and the phenomenon represented by it are identical; words convey power; in fact, the child's fantasy sometimes treats words as omnipotent. To think that someone is dead, to wish him dead, is equivalent to killing him.

Still another characteristic defense mechanism of the obsessive-compulsive neurotic is undoing. He attempts to undo a deed. Contrary to Macbeth who says: "What's done cannot be undone," he follows the notion that: "What is done, *must* be undone." The mechanism of reversal is found in obsessive neurosis but it is not specific for it. The woman who compulsively cleans and scrubs in order to suppress her wish to soil makes use of this mechanism. The warded-off content reappears in the defense.

We shall now turn to the instinctual life of the obsessive-compulsive person. At first glance his sexual life seems free of disturbance. The patient usually reports that he has no complaints in that respect. However, the examiner notices that little value is placed on the emotional aspects of sexual life, and that it is treated not as an expression of tender and erotic feelings, but as a matter of hygiene. Sometimes sexual life is regulated according to a definite system, just as if it were a job like office work. It is evident that the sexual life of these patients is deficient. It is deprived of its emotional content and isolated from affective qualities. It is rationalized and ritualized. The genuine instinctual impulses and the corresponding object relationships are warded off through regression.

We could have treated regression in the context of the defense mechanisms, and also in the context of the ego. The ego regresses too, which is clearly evident in the magical thinking. Regression is still more clearly evident in the area of instinctual life. The subject of regression often presents conceptual difficulties, therefore I intend to treat it in some detail.

First a word in general about defense. Defense is nothing static; the defensive process does not stop with its establishment. For example, the passive-feminine man wards off his passive needs with the help of phallic-narcissistic fantasies. He seeks attention and wants to be admired. This is only the first step in the defense process. The phallic-narcissistic attitude may then be warded off through a general inhibition of activity and enfeeblement of self-assertion. In the end, we see a very timid man. In the course of development defense follows upon defense, each employing its specific mechanism. When we review a life history in psychoanalytic treatment proceeding from the present to the past, we observe the different strata of defenses. To be sure, a complicating factor confuses us. One finds first what one expected to find last. It has been noted repeatedly that "getting soiled" has a particular significance for the obsessive patient. They obviously struggle with anal impulses. Thus one finds first derivatives of the anal phase of development and not the Oedipus complex.

How is this to be explained? The patient regressed, he is frightened by the difficulties of the oedipal phase and retreats to the anal phase. It could also be said that he was pushed back to the anal phase. The Oedipus complex is hidden beneath the anal instinctual strivings and the defenses against them. The patient who is bewildered by the image of the minister and his wife engaged in an act of defecation in church conceals beneath this image guilt feelings and anxieties from the genital phase. When regression has been used as defense, the investigation uncovers first the derivatives from the period to which the regression has proceeded. Sometimes the more infantile instinctual tendencies like the gratification of the anal impulse come to the fore as such. The passive homosexual man employs his anus as a passive organ of sexual pleasure; "sexual" is to be understood here in a broad sense. In such cases we speak of perversions. If the infantile instinctual impulse is warded off the result is a neurosis. The compulsive neurotic wards off anal instinctual impulses with compulsive cleanliness; in turn, these anal impulses had been utilized to keep the oedipal problems out of consciousness. Instinctual life has regressed to the anal stage, and the anal wishes and fantasies are warded off with the help of various mechanisms, such as isolation. Regression invariably recedes to a stage in which difficulties had been experienced. Freud once compared regression with the retreat of a defeated army to old fortified positions. The future compulsive neurotic experienced tension and conflict during the anal phase in connection with his training to cleanliness. Thereby the excretory functions and products acquired an exaggerated significance. The child of the anal phase is not yet clearly aware of the distinction between the sexes. The differentiation into male and female occurs in the phallic phase. Consequently one observes in compulsive neuroses an intensely warded-off bisexuality. The obsessive doubts are often concerned with the question, am I male or female; am I heterosexual or homosexual? I remind you of the example of the pseudo scientific problem of the door: "What is more important, the opening into which the door fits, or the door itself?"

The aggressive drive of the obsessive neurotic patient is no less subject to regressive processes than the libidinal drive. During the anal phase the child begins to discover his independence. He discovers that he can control his sphincters, and that he can hold back or let go some content of his body. This phase has been called the first puberty. When the environment seeks to break the child's awakening will by force, as easily happens in too vigorous toilet training, he develops a stubborn resistance. The aggression of many obsessive neurotics manifests itself in obstinacy. Tormenting of siblings and friends and cruelty to animals also occur in this period. Probably this represents a form of overcoming anxiety: "I am rendered helpless by my parents, but I have power over animals; my parents hurt me, but I am not helpless and dependent, I can hurt others and I am superior to them." In reality the parents need not be cruel at all, they are cruel in the child's fantasy. The fear of fantasied figures is no less painful for the child than the fear of real persons. He cannot yet fully distinguish real from fantasied persons. The childhood obstinacy reappears again in obsessive neurotics, although it is often disguised by apparent docility. They ward off the sadistic form of aggressivity. Obsessive ideas and magical patterns often demonstrate death wishes quite frankly: "If I don't pass the railway crossing before the guard rail is lowered my father will die." The obsessive patient does not act out his aggression directly, his superego prohibits such action.

Freud described a patient who moved a branch lying on the ground aside so that no one would stumble and fall over it. No sooner had he completed this thoughtful action than he felt compelled to take the branch back to its former place. The struggle between hetero- and homosexuality is expressed in obsessive doubts. Fenichel has pointed out that these doubts also express the struggle between aggression and the defense against it.

The anal phase gives rise to certain reactions of jealousy. The child discovers that his products are discarded, while his infant sibling is guarded and loved. Kronfeld (1930) pointed out that the submission of obsessive patients to their compulsions has a quality of addiction. Their instinctual life shows not only sadistic but masochistic traits as well. In the behavior of the obsessive patient the warded-off sadism sometimes becomes evident in peculiar ways. For example, the patient notices a trace of impatience in his doctor and commences a conversation while holding on to the door knob: "I am extremely sorry to have taken so much of your time, but I believe I was justified in doing so, since my condition has grown so much worse. You do not mind my turning to you, do you?" The combination of anxious submission and vexatious behavior is particularly characteristic of obsessive-compulsive neurosis.

We now turn to the ego ideal and the superego of the obsessive neurotic. As a rule the ego ideal's expectations are raised too high, and the superego's demands are too severe and too tyrannical. Carp (1947) called attention to the exaggerated morality of these patients. It is indeed one of their most conspicuous character traits. The superego's severity continues to increase in the course of the patient's life. Bearing in mind the genesis of the superego one can readily imagine the consequences of its mounting severity. The oedipal phase has been difficult. The failure to integrate it resulted in a regression. However, the impulses of the anal phase are no less forbidden than those of the oedipal period, and the superego condemns them just as strictly. Occasional indulgence of the anal impulses induces the superego to impose stern punishment on the ego. The parents have become a part of the person's superego and this parental derivative is no less intolerant of the libidinal and aggressive impulses of the anal stage than the parents were. Often the superego is much stricter than the parents were. The relations between superego and ego represent the continuation of the relations between parent and child. The child stubbornly resisted the paternal prohibitions. Similarly, he resists the superego prohibitions, without being aware of their source. "Beware," says the superego. The ego attempts to defend itself against the superego's threats, but its fears of the superego are so intense that it feels compelled to give in. The ego's fear of becoming soiled further contributes to its helplessness. The parents seldom were as harsh in their treatment of the children as the superego is towards the ego. The projected hostility of the child makes the parents appear hostile and threatening. Moreover, the patients turn their hostile feelings against the self, and assail themselves with prohibitions, self-condemnatory reproaches and self-punitive attitudes. At times the ego is helplessly tossed about between the insistent instinctual urges and the sadistic superego. In such a situation the patient is driven to despair. He particularly attempts to placate his superego after having given in to the drive. He behaves like the members of primitive cultures who seek to propitiate the evil spirits with various offerings. Freud ascribed the fact that obsessive patients, unlike those with depression, are not suicidal to the circumstance that not all of the available psychic energy is involved in their conflict. Nevertheless the patient suffers intensely. Fenichel has aptly called his struggles with the sadistic superego and with the infantile instinctual impulses an inner two-front war. In some cases the ego is almost entirely taken over by the two antagonists and retains only very little energy for adaptation.

At times the ego attempts to deceive its superego and assumes an attitude of obedience to its commands, while in fact giving in to the instinctual impulses. In this fashion the struggle with the parents characteristic of the anal period is carried on in the neurosis.

Our next subject is the relation between symptom and character in obsessive-compulsive neuroses. The previously described familiar criterion is of little help. A compulsion is ego-alien by definition; one can designate the character type commonly found among obsessive patients a compulsive character. Many people have habits which are very much like compulsive phenomena, for instance adherence to certain rituals and exaggerated orderliness. We became acquainted with typical character traits of obsessive neurotic persons when we discussed their ego functions, their conscience and their instinctual life. Excessive morality, ambivalence, the inclination to rationalization, intellectualization, isolation, and reversal all contribute to the formation of the typical compulsive character.

There are, of course, more than one form of compulsive

character. Freud (1908) described a form of character based on regression to the anal stage and marked by the characteristic triad of orderliness, parsimony and obstinacy. According to Freud, the orderliness refers to "bodily cleanliness as well as conscientiousness in carrying out small duties and trustworthiness. . . . Parsimony may appear in the exaggerated form of avarice; and obstinacy can go over into defiance . . ." (p. 169).

The subject of parsimony takes us to the connection between feces and money, a topic which evokes merriment in some people, resistance in others, and in still others, both reactions. Feces is one of the first products of man. The child has a certain power over producing or withholding feces. The excrements come of his body and are experienced as his possession. He can part with them willingly, offer them to those he favors as a sign of his affection, and he can also withhold them and thereby demonstrate his power. Much of what we just described is equally valid for money. Money can be amassed, saved, and then suddenly spent. In many persons the libidinal significance of these actions by far surpasses their practical significance. We may assume that ancient drive gratifications are participating in the person's management of money. The secretiveness of most people in money matters is of interest. One is reminded of the expression *pecunia non olet* and of the story of the donkey defecating golden ducats.

Obstinacy is a continuation of the child's resistance to training in the anal phase; orderliness is a consquence of the child's obedience to introjected parents.

The work of Freud mentioned above had tremendous significance for the development of a scientific characterology. Before its appearance character was viewed as innate, and characterology was mainly concerned with classification. Freud arrived at a dynamic and functional conceptualization of character. He perceived it as a habitual adaptation to the external and inner world. Character must be considered in relation to the infantile drives. It is not something static and unchanging. It is a meaningful response to the situation in which the child develops and grows. Freud (1908, p. 175) says that permanent character traits are either unchanged extensions of the original instinctual impulses, sublimations of those impulses, or reaction formations against them.

It is not always easy to recognize the character forms connected with regression to the anal phase. Generally when examining the character of patients with compulsive symptoms one discovers anal character traits, but these traits may appear without symptoms of an obsessive-compulsive neurosis. The anal character may be present in a very disguised form. In certain situations it becomes evident that the anal character functions like a cloak of armor which impedes the person's inner mobility. Parsimony, obstinacy and orderliness are fairly conspicuous traits. In many people, the manifestations of the anal character neurosis are subtle and inconspicuous. Thus they may impress us by their seemingly excellent adaptation. They never fail, and are held out as exemplary models to be emulated. However, they are inadequate in situations in which it is important to experience and display genuine emotion. We are familiar with such persons in our environment. They appear impeccably attired, they are neat and always cleanly shaven; the women of this type are invariably well-dressed, but their clothes lack imagination and are often not tastefully chosen. These people are not conspicuously parsimonious. They can be generous, but they have great difficulties in giving when it is expected of them. Concealed by their apparent mildness is an obstinacy no less intense than that of people with openly displayed anal characteristic traits. In fact their obstinacy appears even more unyielding than the frankly acted out stubbornness. If they are reproached for injustices resulting from their attitude, they defend themselves with arguments to prove that they are correct. They act as if they personified justice itself, and those who reproach them will end up feeling that they had been unfair and wrong. Sometimes they appear to yield and acknowledge the justification of the reproach, yet they remain unchanged and continue to follow their own path. Their married life is indifferent because of their lack of spontaneity. They frequently derive a hidden pleasure from not too risky gambles. They speculate cautiously with modest amounts of money and secretly enjoy their possessions. Not only are they unable to give when it is expected of them, they also cannot permit others to give to them. To accept a gift means to be passive, and to be passive means to be feminine. A significant factor in the inability to receive is the fear of losing their independence and having no will of their own.

The manner in which these people manage time is worthy of note. It is difficult for them to change their plans. To arrive late is a horror, and worse still is to leave late. They abruptly interrupt important functions or conversations in order to proceed with the activity they had scheduled. They do everything at a strictly specified time. One cannot escape the impression that they repeat the childhood situation in which they related to the mother with a determined expression of their will: "I shall empty my bowels when I want to, no sooner and no later." They obey the letter of the law and justify failures this way. These people are often dogmatic and peremptory in their views and attitudes. They almost always refuse to accept someone else's opinion. The meaning is not the same as in the phallic-narcissistic type of opinionated and arbitrary behavior. The latter tends to brag about his knowledge, and to impose his wisdom on everybody within earshot. The dogmatism of the anal character is not so much concerned with displaying his own superior knowledge as with the need to reject that of others. The primary motivation for the self-righteousness of the phallic-narcissistic type is pride, and for that of the anal character the desire to reject the values of others.

Another character type related to obsessive neurosis systematizes life. The favorite defense mechanisms of these people are rationalization and intellectualization. People of this type need not be greedy, thrifty, orderly, or well-groomed; however, they lack spontaneity. These devotees of a systematic life have a closed world image, never experiencing surprises, expecting nothing new in life, everything that can possibly happen in life is provided for in their system and is regulated in accordance with a prearranged plan. Their rationalizing has the same quality as the thought processes of obsessive neurotic patients; the rationalizations are magical and far from being realistic. These people have keen judgment in many areas, yet they can also waste much time discussing the relative merits of various diets and prescriptions for a wholesome life. By means of rationalization and systematization all real experience is kept away from consciousness; thinking is employed not so much in the service of establishing connections in reality, but rather in the service of escape from reality. They are also passionate classifiers. Freud (1926) remarked on this subject as follows:

> To order the unknown according to known categories is the task of science. Compulsive systematizing, performed not for the purpose of mastering reality but rather in order to deny certain aspects of it, falsifying reality, is a caricature of science.

The regulation of life according to a predetermined system is found among some religious groups. The faith of these people impresses those outside the group not so much as belief in God, but rather as a boundless faith in their own system. In our present society many of the above-described character traits are highly valued; their owners are praised as decent, good people. The neurotic systematizers are often respected as philosophical thinkers. The poverty of emotional experience of these people seems to escape the observer's attention.

Evaluation of obsessive neuroses and obsessive characters must take into consideration the cultural and social setting of the patient. In keeping with our functional and dynamic approach we have to consider whether adapted functioning is still possible, or whether the person is totally overwhelmed by his compulsions. The more advanced stages of obsessive neurosis greatly impede the ability of the patient to function as a productive member of society. Small wonder that obsessive-compulsive neurosis is considered by some to be an entity between neurosis and psychosis. There are indeed cases of obsessive neurosis severe enough to warrant, even to require care in a psychiatric hospital. In very severe cases of obsessive neurosis the differential diagnosis of schizophrenia must be considered. Even those cases in which the patients manage to stay on in their homes are not without serious difficulties. For example: A young patient is constantly compelled to separate objects from each other. He is particularly concerned that his parents' shoes do not touch. When he finds the shoes in close proximity, he addresses his parents with passionate reproaches: "If you were truly interested in me, you would show me more consideration." His brother-in-law who lives in the same household thinks the parents should pay no attention to the boy's peculiarities. This same boy loves animals. He picks up his sister's dog, strokes it affectionately and then kicks it. The sister notices this and takes the dog from him, to his great consternation. The phenomenon of the war on two fronts is particulary distinct here. He feels called upon to struggle against moral decay, he wants to be a good example, chaste and pure, and he worries his analyst because he is tormented by the compulsive impulse to cut off his penis with a razor. He also sees himself as tragic hero in opposition to the sexual norms and prejudices of middle class society. When his therapist discusses his masturbation conflicts he accuses the therapist of wanting to seduce him, of being an ally of his drives. At the same time he experiences the analyst as a stern judge who condemns him. He attempts again and again to involve his therapist in discussions of philosophy and of *Weltanschauung.* Owing to his superior intelligence his school work is adequate though it is impaired by his conflicts with authority. School work provides him with some satisfactions. His compulsive activities and his fear of soiling himself brought much hardship to the family; nevertheless it was possible to avoid his placement in an institution. In his case psychoanalytic treatment had to be combined with measures designed to give his whole family some insight.

Compulsive manifestations are related not only to anal but also to genital impulses. Regression is not always massive and clearly evident. The compulsion sometimes is limited to a single area of the person's experience. One of my female patients had the compulsive impulse to put her little son to death. This impulse occurred only when she saw a bread knife. Although this was the only manifestation of her compulsive neurosis the condition was exceedingly painful. Though she had other neurotic symptoms they were not compulsive in nature.

Frequently compulsive neuroses are coupled with phobic symptoms. The reverse is less common. Even when a phobic manifestation has a clearly anal significance it need not become a compulsive phenomenon. Other phobias such as claustrophobia, agoraphobia and fear of heights are seldom accompanied by compulsive phenomena. To avoid open spaces out of fear is not compulsive, since such an avoidance does not meet the criterion of a compulsive condition, i.e., it is not subjectively experienced as an irresistible compulsion. One can observe phobic phenomena in compulsive characters, yet it is advisable to differentiate the phobic from the compulsive character. Bastiaans (1957) noted that the phobic character intends to avoid a previously desired situation. In the phobic character an ego-alien phobic symptom becomes ego-syntonic.

As we have seen there are considerable differences between the hysterical and compulsive characters. There are of course neuroses in which both hysterical and compulsive characteristics occur simultaneously.

In clinical discussions one sometimes hears the opinion that the obsessive-compulsive neurosis is in fact a depression which becomes manifest as a compulsive neurosis. This view is not tenable, although the simultaneous occurrence of depressive and compulsive symptoms is not unusual. A severe superego, introjected aggression and thwarted drives with passive aims easily cause depressive conditions. The compulsive neurosis may run its course in stages of different intensity, and an endogenous factor may contribute one of the causes of this uneven course. Yet, these possibilities are not suficient reasons for saying that the compulsive neurosis is "really a depression." The inclination to make the diagnosis of depression may be determined by the wish to use electric shock. This kind of treatment may avoid confrontation with the difficult problems of the patient and with one's own lack of insight. When a neurosis progresses unfavorably and does not respond to therapeutic measures, some psychiatrists feel impelled to declare that the patient's condition is really a schizophrenic illness. A diagnosis should be made on the basis of the manifest symptomatology and not on the basis of unverified conjecture. One cannot deduce the diagnosis of schizophrenia from the presence of a neurosis. Inaccurate diagnostic work should not be condoned. Only once in my practice did it prove to be extraordinarily difficult to make a differential diagnosis. Such a contingency occurs only in the most seriously ill cases. The difficulty may be compounded by the tendency of the compulsive neurotic to rationalize and ward off his affects. In some cases one indeed wonders whether what one observes is the flattening of affect of the schizophrenic. Compulsive symptoms do occur in schizophrenia, in depressions, and in epilepsy as well. They also occur in the syndrome of hypersensitivity, and in postpartum emotional disturbances. Generally a diminished integrative capacity, regardless of its souce, may cause latent neurotic problems to become manifest.

A word about the relation between compulsive and psychasthenic conditions. Bastiaans (1957) is of the opinion that psychasthenia represents a variant of the obsessive-compulsive character. He believes that the defense against passive-feminine needs is the main dynamic factor in psychasthenia, whereas defense against sadistic impulses is central in compulsive characters. Is there a constitutional predisposition to obsessional neuroses? If so, is it identical with the predisposition to psychasthenia? That illness is characterized by tics, phobic and obsessional manifestations and an *abaissement du niveau mental*. Indeed it seems that some constitutions predispose the person to the development of neuroses though there is no certainty in the matter. It is difficult to determine whether psychasthenia actually is the constitutional matrix for the obsessive-compulsive neuroses. It is preferable to assume that a combination of factors, constitutional and environmental, may result in the development of either neurosis or psychasthenia. One may also assume that these factors include the person's temperament, and the scope and availability of his psychic energy. The evaluation of the relative importance of the different factors is of paramount importance. It is obvious that one cannot expect cure from the resolution of unconscious conflicts when the pathological condition is largely based on a constitutional deficiency.

Related to neurasthenia and psychasthenia is the condition described as asthenia. The patient's complaints are expressions of weakness and fatigue-ability rather than of intrapsychic tensions. Such people indeed give the impression of asthenia, i.e., lack of strength. In evaluating asthenia one must bear in mind that fatigue may be the result of a constitutional deficiency, and also of faulty utilization of energy. This is the case when powerful instinctual impulses must be kept unconscious by equally powerful defenses. This can be compared to two train engines pushing against each other with equal power. The result is a standstill. The differentiation is not always easy. That the efficacy of the psychic functions diminishes in conditions of exhaustion of the nervous system is well known. We can observe it readily in certain conditions, as for instance in the syndrome of emotional hypersensitivity.

In regard to the course of obsessive-compulsive conditions it may be said that some cases are transient, though on the whole their course is less capricious than the course of other neuroses. Adolescence and the menopausal age are susceptible periods. Obsessive manifestations often begin in adolescence. At first diffuse anxiety makes its appearance, and phobic or neurasthenic symptoms may herald the outbreak of an obsessive illness. Sometimes long periods of remission occur. The patients often ascribe the precipitating fact to seemingly minor events. Situations which mobilize the need for defense against aggressive or sadomasochistic anal impulses, for instance, the witnessing of a bloody accident may precipitate the outbreak of the compulsive neurosis. Where the obsessive manifestation occurs as a symptom of a schizophrenic or depressive psychosis, the course will naturally depend on the dominant illness. In all these instances a careful differential diagnosis is indispensable.

Freud ascribed the predisposition to obsessional neurosis to constitutional factors and a fixation to the anal stage of development. Fixations occur when too little or too much gratification has been experienced at a given stage. Particular significance is ascribed to deliberate and unexpected changes in the attitude of the parents to the child's needs. No obsessional neurosis comes into being, however, without preceding difficulties in the assimilation of sexual and aggressive impulses connected with the Oedipus complex. Many compulsions do not have an anal, pregenital content, but are derivatives of phallic sexual impulses. Nevertheless, there invariably occurs a regression to an earlier period of libidinal development, a retreat from phallic sexuality which is overburdened with guilt and castration fears. Besides being a retreat from phallic sexuality the regression is simultaneously a return to anal impulses and gratifications. This defense impairs the functions of the ego, reality is misread because of the ensuing isolation and denial of some aspects of reality. The synthetic function of the ego fails, and the neurosis develops. The fixation accounts for the possibility of the regression. It is determined by the child's innate qualities and by the attitude of his parents. A natural process which, if paid less attention, would result in the child's spontaneous control of his sphincters, becomes a battle for cleanliness which many mothers conduct like a holy war, whose victims, unfortunately, are the child's spontaneity and happiness.

We have reached the discussion of the social and cultural behavior models which dominate child rearing. When demands are made of the young child which he is unable to fulfill, he is confused and bewildered by them. Feces placed in a certain receptacle are enthusiastically praised, yet the same feces at another place are an object of the mother's loathing and anger. How should the child integrate these contradictory impressions. It is not astonishing that his resistance and rebelliousness are thus evoked. The child learns to control a physiological function, i.e., to hold onto or to give up his excrements. To his own surprise he discovers that he can produce something that is his own, having emerged from his body. The child reacts with helpless rage when he is subjected to enemas, (the prototype of a rape) and forced to lose something. This loss is accompanied by powerful and irritating sensations, while the voluntary production of his feces is experienced pleasurably. The mother who hitherto supplied warmth and security, now causes pain and displeasure. The aura of confidence and trust vanishes and the anger which takes over can create a concept of a world which wants to deprive the person of all things he wants to keep for himself. The struggle about cleanliness occurs in the developmental stage in which the child discovers his own will power and his relative independence of the environment. If the child is subjected to the parental will too much during this period, having a will of one's own easily becomes being obstinate. If in addition to being subjected to ambitious toilet training the child's inclination to smear and mess is also prohibited without providing him with opportunities for sublimation, he reacts with particularly violent protestations and with pathological development.

The mother of one of my patients, a well meaning but distressed woman, reacted with panic and horror when her little daughter, my patient in her later life, overturned a cup of milk, blew soap bubbles, etc. The child reacted with an obsessive defiance which later became a prevailing intrapsychic attitude. She could not carry out her own decisions, she wanted to work but could not. The early struggles with the mother later became a chronic dispute with an internalized object. The image of the little child on the pot who annoys her mother by her disobedience is perhaps amusing. The later consequences of this disagreement may be less amusing. The opposition against oneself is a very painful symptom, it is in fact one of the most tormenting complaints. To be neat and orderly has a double significance in our society. It is wrong to underestimate the social and cultural influences which support mothers in their outdated attitudes. The pretty and clean dress of the little girl is evidence of the good care the mother gives her child, and it is also a status symbol. It signifies that "this nice child comes from a superior family." I recently observed the following scene: From my window I see a neighborhood with many new homes and many children. It has been raining and the ground is wet. The blue sky is reflected in the puddles. Some boys lash at the water with sticks and branches enjoying themselves immensely. Their father looks on and smiles. A little girl plays in the mud, her face shows streaks of dirt, and she glows with pleasure. Little Yvonne stands nearby and looks on with disapproval. Her childish face shows an expression of moral superiority, and is already marred by an air of arrogance. She is wearing a cream colored formal little dress with pink flowers and a huge bow. "Yvonne," calls her mother, "step away from the puddle, quick, think of your pretty dress, the children will spray you with mud." Yvonne moves to the side and bumps into a little girl who awkwardly maneuvers her tricycle. Yvonne angrily gives her a strong push, the child's tricycle rolls off the sidewalk, the child falls and cuts her lip. Little Yvonne, having displaced and vented her anger at her mother, appears defiantly content.

On the occasion of this child's visit to our home some time ago, we heard her discourse in this fashion: "That father of Gerd has such a crazy mustache. Mother says, these people have no car and money. They are crazy, I don't want to go to Gerd's birthday party, and I don't like his playing in the mud puddles. . . ." She ridicules a little boy who limps and drags his leg because of a nerve injury.

This little girl has begun to turn into the full-fledged elegant matron she will be one day, given to gossiping and slandering. She will be a woman concerned mainly with social status, seeking to belong to the "best" circles. She will always exhort her husband to earn more money. She will be more interested in success than in happiness, more interested in appearance and pretentiousness than in meaningful or useful activities. She will resent those who can enjoy life spontaneously. Her parents, who consider themselves among the "better" people, have made an early start in making her into such a person.

Menninger (1943) formulated it thus: "The emphasis on production, the value of time, the importance of material possessions, the striving for wealth and its implied power, are all paramount goals in our age of civilization, which might be said to be in anal phase" (p. 61).

Children in our society are taught to be "nice," neat and orderly and to renounce the pleasure which their physiological functions provide. They are to be "nice" in a double sense, not "dirty" as regards their bodies, and approved by a society in which to be nice and orderly is valued more highly than concern for others and reverence for life.

The basis for sexual inhibitions is prepared during the anal phase. The concept "pure" thus has the additional meaning of "asexual." It is as if the qualities of being clean, and asexual were mankind's most precious properties.

Psychiatry is of great importance in the education of our children. A sober appraisal of compulsive-obsessive disturbances stimulates us to look to preventive psychiatry. Compulsive neurosis is a serious illness which causes much grief, and compulsive-obsessive anal attitudes are detrimental for the development of our culture. The rejection of one's body, the dearth of gratifications evoke aggression, which seeks an outlet in hate, envy, and the lust for war. Instead of love and kindness, excessive order, miserliness and obstinacy proliferate in abundance.

8

———⊃∞∞CCᴼᴼᴼᴼᴼᴼᴼᴼᴼᴼᴼ⊂———

ORAL CHARACTER,
DEPRESSION AND ADDICTION

It is logical to classify neurotic disturbances from the standpoint of the development of the personality. Yet, one encounters difficulties in this attempt.

In the case of obsessive neurosis we observed that although anal impulses lent a specific character to the illness, the activation of these impulses was a result of regression. The concept of regression is of fundamental significance for the understanding of the neurotic disorders. The child, being unable to resolve the problems of the oedipal stage owing to castration fears and guilt feelings, seeks to escape these problems by giving up the genital position and falling back to an earlier developmental stage.

We find confirmation from Freud's formulation that the Oedipus complex is the nucleus of the neurosis. Whenever we probe more deeply into the structure of obsessive neurotic problems we encounter unresolved oedipal problems concealed by anal impulses and the defenses against them.

In classifying the neuroses in groups connected with the oral, anal and oedipal phases one must bear in mind that the appearance of problems connected with one phase may represent a defense against problems from another phase. In addition we must not lose sight of the organic continuity of the phases. They are not isolated from one another like the

207

stations on a railway line. It invariably depends on the manner of resolution of the earlier phases whether or not the person is sufficiently prepared to weather the difficulties of the next stage of development. Difficulties in adaptation related to an earlier developmental stage can readily be activated by disturbances of a later stage.

In depression, addiction and some forms of character neurosis we observe psychic processes which belong to the oral phase of libidinal development. The patient has either never developed beyond that stage, or has regressed to it. We must not forget that the regression involves not only the instinctual life, but also the ego. Different mechanisms of the ego's regression occur. The ego may regress because of pressure from the environment, or because of an insoluble instinctual conflict, i.e., the regression serves to avoid oedipal problems. Indisputably, the Oedipus complex is the nucleus of the neurosis.

There is a gradual transition between the two regressive phenomena mentioned above. They are determined by the person's constitution and by his experiences in the first years of life. Regression to the oral phase is the matrix for the depressions and addictions. This means more than acquisition of an oral pattern in instinctual life. The oral stage involves much more than its name indicates. In this first stage the skin is as much an erogenous zone as the mouth. The desire for warmth and security equals in importance the need for oral gratification. Harlow's experiments clearly demonstrate these propositions. He raised young monkeys with two kinds of dummy mother surrogates: one, made of wire, had nursing bottles attached; the other had wire covered with soft cloth but no bottles. The baby monkeys nursed at the bottles but then promptly ran to and clutched at the soft and warm cloth "mother." If they were frightened while both dummies were in the cage, they fled to the cloth covered dummy. If only the "oral" wire dummy was present they became panicky. Its presence completely failed to reassure them.

In speaking of the oral phase we apply the concept in its broad sense; we consider all aspects of the instinctual needs and also the ego development corresponding to that phase. The skin sensations and the experience of warmth are no less important in this phase than the feeling of satiation and the sensations in the mucous membrance of the mouth. It is noteworthy that the sense of security was provided by the warm and soft dummy. In spite of this "mother" being unable to supply it with food, or to protect it, the little monkey seems to react as if it received protection and security from this "pseudo mother." In one experiment a mechanical Teddy bear was introduced into the cage. This toy could be made to move about and beat its drum. The frightened little monkeys fled to the cloth dummy, hid their faces in the terry cloth and clung to it. They seemed to derive comfort and courage from this contact; they began to watch the toy bear and even to venture forward curiously in its direction. They used the cloth "mother" as their operational base. It is not different in the case of human children. The mother provides the child with a feeling of security, which enables him to undertake actions increasing in scope, and to explore the world around him. The very young child requires such a "symbiotic" relationship in order to grow without impairment of his personality. Regression to this stage implies a longing for such symbiosis.

The young child is dependent on his mother for the gratification of his instinctual needs; at the same time she enhances his self-esteem with her attitude of encouragement. He feels helpless and frustrated in her absence. Libidinal and narcissistic gratifications at this time coincide. The insight into these circumstances is indispensable for the understanding of the depressive conditions. The loss of love or the loss of a love object invariably causes a profound injury to the depressive person's self-esteem and self-confidence.

People with a so-called oral character are excessively dependent on love and expressions of love. They are also very demanding. Their frustration tolerance is low. What the average adult experiences as a minor disappointment, these people perceive as a bitter frustration, as an injury difficult to overcome. Many of them tend to act out the feelings generated by their frustration. They seek to receive their "love nourishment" from as many people as possible. They do not see the individual person in others, but merely suppliers of gratification. We say, their objects are need-satisfying. At times these people become pathologically attached to one person. Often persons with an oral character assume an overindulgent attitude to others, in which case their own dependent and demanding pattern is less conspicuous. In such a setting they relate to their partner in the way in which they themselves wish to be treated. A mutual mother-child relationship develops between them. They appear more capable of object-love than they are in reality. Sometimes they seek to bribe others with the expressions of their love. There are no absolute criteria to distinguish these people from those who are truly adult. The distinctions are only relative. The person capable of adult and mature love, to some degree loves himself, but this component of his love is not as pervasive as in oral characters. Unlike the latter, he is capable of considering and attending to the needs of his partner.

NEUROTIC DEPRESSIONS

Depressive reactions occur in many neuroses. When a mood of dejection is the main symptom of the disorder we call it a depression, when that mood coincides with other more predominant pathologic manifestations we refer to it as depressive reaction.

Neurotic patients react depressively to many different symptoms. Thwarting of instinctual needs results in a feeling of discontent; the resulting aggression is incapable of direct expression and turns inward against the self. Masturbation

conflicts of adolescence offer an occasion to study the genesis
of depressive reactions. The series of psychic events leading
to a depressed mood is as follows: Fear of sexuality, resentment about the frustration; owing to guilt feelings the resentment cannot be expressed; general discouragement because
of the ego's inability to either gratify or silence the demands
of the drive; hypochondriacal and paranoid responses to the
guilt feelings.

The frustration of the need to be loved, and of the drives
with a passive aim is particularly instrumental in the development of the more conspicuous depressive conditions. The
frustration of these needs awakens aggression, which cannot
be expressed owing to the fear of losing the love object, and
is therefore turned against the self. The patient is unable to
break out of the vicious circle. In addition he experiences
resentment about the dejected mood itself. We must not
underestimate the extent and significance of this feeling.
"Life holds nothing for me; others enjoy life, for me it is
nothing but a heavy burden."

We shall proceed to examine the psychic mechanisms of
depression. The superego of depressive people is excessively
severe and punitive. It appropriates the resentment which
originally was felt towards others and directs it against the
self. "I am furious and want to revenge myself on others" is
turned into "my conscience rages against me." The severe
conscience imposes new frustrations. These provoke aggression, which again is blocked. All too frequently this process
ends in a wild outburst of rage against the self. Neurotic
depressives are by no means immune from suicide. An element of revenge is sometimes clearly discernible. By means
of his dejected attitude the patient says to others: "See what
you have done to me." The feelings of guilt—"I am so mean
to others"—frequently signify also "others are so mean to
me." "I kill myself" often implies "you have killed me."
When the histrionic element in this attitude predominates

we speak of a hysterical depression. Let us review the role of the ego and its functions in depressions. In cases in which pathological gloom is the central and not a concomitant symptom, regression invariably determines the nature of the condition.

Frustration of drives with passive aims sharply lowers the self-esteem which depends entirely on expressions of love from others. A depressed patient can no more free himself from a frustrating relationship than an infant can declare himself independent of his mother. The depressed patient regularly attracts the unfriendly attention of superiors. He is unable to break with an unfaithful mistress because his ego can function only in a symbiotic relationship. One of my female patients expressed it in the following words: "I cannot admire the swans and sea gulls when I am alone; I cannot enjoy anything without enjoying it with someone." At certain times this feeling is familiar to all of us, for instance, during an intense period of being in love. The depressive is a chronically disappointed lover who never ceases to be in love. The self-esteem of the depressed person and his adaptive functions depend on the presence of another person with whom he entertains a symbiotic relationship.

One should not consider the inclination to form dependent symbiotic relationships without considering the aggression turned inward resulting from it. The trait of wanting everything from the other person makes frustrations inescapable. Each episode of unhappiness is experienced as a refusal by the person on whom the patient depends and whom he perceives as an omnipotent figure capable of granting or refusing happiness.

Disturbances of ego functions in depressions are closely connected with instinctual problems. In this context we have to discuss "malignant regression," which is one of the least malleable subjects of psychoanalytic theory. Briefly formulated, the theory claims that depression is the result of rage at an introjected object. We shall attempt to clarify this at first rather puzzling formulation. We have already pointed out in the discussion of guilt feelings and self-recriminations of depressed patients that these self-recriminations in reality seem to be accusations of others, and that the suicidal attempt appears to be a simultaneous attempt at homicide. We stressed this observation in connection with the discussion of suicide, always a danger in severe depressions. Many researchers have noted a reproachful attitude and a revenge wish in hysterical depressions. But it was Freud who discovered that the self-recriminations are accusations of others in nonhysterical depressions as well, and that suicide is psychologically a form of homicide. Phenomenologically the hysterical and the depressive self-accusations have little in common. The wish of the hysterical patient to attack someone else with his misery is easily recognizable. In fact this wish is not infrequently quite close to consciousness. The guilt feelings and suicidal ideas of the depressive patient have a much more intense quality. These patients do not act in accordance with their environment. Their depressive experience takes place much more intrapsychically than that of the hysterical patient. The depressive patient is immersed within himself, while the hysteric pleads with the environment. Nevertheless the self-reproaches of the depressive patient are also reproaches against others, and his suicide is most certainly also a homicidal attempt. A decisive factor in these cases is the malignant regression and the introjection of the love object into the ego. The depressive patient wants to do away with the introjected object within himself. At this point the reader is likely to think that Freud went too far, or that the matter has become too complicated for his taste.

Let us review a clinical example:

A son loses his father, or an assistant loses a respected boss. At the memorial services sentiments like the following are voiced: "We shall continue to follow in his footsteps," "We shall endeavor to continue the work begun by him, and emulate his example." Such expressions are often nothing but empty phrases. Yet, it is true that we identify with the deceased. One also hears reactions to loss like these: "It is as if he continued to exist in me, as if I have taken him into my heart, he lives in me." When we try to imagine graphically these ideas we begin to understand what introjection implies. The other person has become part of us. Let us now imagine that we are furious at the other person, that we have introjected not a loved but a hated person, and that we passionately desire to express our rage against this person. The depressed person does just that. He rages against the hated figure within himself; that is the crucial issue. The essential element of malignant regression is the taking into oneself of the hated object. A precondition of this type of regression is a very strong emotional attachment to the introjected object. To be linked to a person so intensely that one cannot do without him, and to hate and bitterly reproach him at the same time, is one of the most painful forms of ambivalence. We know that all depressions are intimately connected with ambivalent feelings, and that these feelings are precipitated by disappointment in the loved object.

Why do we describe this reaction pattern as a regression? What is the connection between the introjection of an ambivalently experienced object and regression?

I shall begin by quoting a patient who has been abandoned by his mistress: "It is now two and one half years since she left me, and it seems like yesterday. I cannot free myself from her. She was so mean to me, she hurt me and humiliated me, and yet we also had such happy times together. Reason tells me that we could not have stayed happy for very long. Yet I think of her constantly, her image is in the background of everything I experience. My first thought when I wake up in the morning is of her; it is as if she was in me. Why don't I kill her or kill her child? Would that help me?" These expressions illustrate clearly the man's intense bondage as well as his bitter anger.

The growth of personality in early childhood takes place by way of the child's taking in and assimilating the impressions he receives from the mother, like the body takes in the food and builds its own substance out of it. When regression occurs these primitive forms of human relationships, like the taking into oneself, replace the more mature patterns, in which the ego is separated from others by more clearly defined boundaries. Just as we can introduce into our body noxious substances, so we can incorporate into our psyche something which is damaging and even destructive to us. We must not forget that body and psyche are not two separate things but form a unit. Some depressed people complain about "something bad and dangerous" within them. Language takes cognizance of the unity of body and soul when it uses expressions like: "I cannot stomach this man," or "this is an unpalatable idea." When we have incorporated something into our personality that we want to destroy, its destruction can be accomplished only by destroying ourselves. The pleasurable enactment of the aggressive impulse against the other person becomes self-destruction. A patient wrote to me as follows: "I imagine how the wheels of the railroad engine will tear my sick head from my body that does not want to die. I should smash my head on the rock." This patient's treatment demonstrated that she was filled with a passionate infantile hatred of her husband, and that in childhood she hated her mother with equal intensity.

To summarize: Malignant regression occurs when the patient's neurotic conflicts force him to regress to an early infantile position. There are as yet no genuine object relations. At this time, the child is building up his self through incorporation and introjection. We call the regression malignant because the object which has evoked the child's rage is introjected and becomes part of the self, and the child's rage attacks the object within the self.

Intense bonds between people are always accompanied to some degree by processes of introjection. It is certainly the case in married couples: Think of the common observation how much alike partners can become in the course of their marriage. It is helpful to use the concept of symbiosis for our understanding of depressive processes. This concept is probably easier to comprehend than introjection.

The infant lives in a symbiotic relationship with his mother. The psychological boundary between his ego and the mother has not yet been established. When regression to this early phase takes place the need for such a symbiotic relationship is revived. In certain situations the wish to return to the security and safety of this primary unity is reactivated. If the person with whom such a union is sought thwarts that longing the resulting rage is directed both against the self and the thwarting person. Insofar as one lives in the situation described as "I and the other person are one" hate of the other becomes self-hate. It need not astound us that patients in this situation commit murder and suicide. Superficially the suicide that follows the murder appears to be an expression of fear of the unavoidable punishment or atonement. The deeper motive is the wish to murder the other in oneself, and oneself in the other. The fact that not hatred alone but an ambivalent set of feelings cause such a deed of desperation becomes clearly evident in the wishful fantasy that in death the two will become inseparably reunited. In cases where the suicidal attempt fails this fantasy can often be recovered. In these instances the aggression has found its way to action. However, that is not the typical depressive position. One finds episodes of murder and suicide in patients driven to despair and frenzy by their pathological jealousy. In typical depression the aggression is turned inward and the patient's fury rages intrapsychically.

The patient I have quoted before described his lady friend as a heavenly angel. Inquiring in detail what she offered him did not reveal too much evidence of her affection. Since her sexuality was neurotically exaggerated one could not ascribe the sexual gratification which he received to her affection for him. Nevertheless he perceived her willingness as proof of love. He considered the disappointments and cruelties she had inflicted on him as entirely his own fault. He quite incorrectly ascribed to her an attitude similar to his own readiness to sacrifice everything in her behalf. In this symbiosis he became dark as the night, and she as radiant as the sun. It required much effort to make it clear to him that he had loved a creation of his fantasy who became all the more beautiful the more he condemned himself. He had loved a fantasied image that was part of himself. While the distrustful person sees only the worst in others and the best in himself, many depressed patients react in the opposite sense. To them others are perfect, while they are worthless and do not merit receiving love and affection. Why do depressed people react in this way? After all, the manner in which the distrustful person distorts reality, i.e., by projecting his hostility, is not as dangerous to life as the acting out of aggression against the self. Depressed patients can no more openly resent the person who disappoints them than the infant can openly resent the mother, who is the bearer of everything good, of safety, peace, fulfillment and security.

Richard Wagner put in poetic words the sensations of the desperate, lonely and helpless infant when he sees the mother's smiling face approach him again:

Auf wonniger Blumen
lichten Wogen
kommt wie sanft
ans Land gezogen.
Sie lächelt mir Trost
und süsse Ruh,
sie führt mir letzte
Labung zu . . .

On waves of flowers
lightly lifted,
gently toward
the land she has drifted.
Her smile brings me ease
and sweet repose:
One last relief
she on me bestows . . .

Little Tristan in his crib cannot be angry with his heavenly
Isolde, he is much too fearful of losing her, and even more
fearful of destroying her with his anger. He is furious with
her but the fury rages against his own self.

We have seen that the frustration of preoedipal wishes and
the inhibition of aggression is based on several factors. Since
they act in common, psychiatric usage fails to separate them.
An attempt to differentiate these factors is nevertheless clari-
fying and helpful for the diagnosis. Inhibition can signify that
the hostility intended for someone else has been turned on
one's own ego after differentiation between ego and external
world has taken place. This mechanism is present in many
neuroses which conform in their structure and dynamics to
the hysterical neuroses. It is a disturbance of the relation of
the ego to the drive, characterized by an insufficient defense.
It is comparable to repression which usually accompanies
this mechanism. But that is not what we term malignant
regression.

In malignant regression the ego is affected as well. A hated
object becomes a part of the ego and the hostility turns
against it. One can compare the first instance to bombs falling on friendly territory instead of on hostile territory. The
second case can be compared to civil war.

In malignant regression the ego acquires an aspect of bad-
ness and hostility. It is important to differentiate between the
two mechanisms of introjection of a hated object and turning
of aggression against the self.

In the therapy of depressed patients one must determine which factor contributes most to their dejection. In many cases it is the quest for the symbiotic relationship. These depressions manifest themselves as a nostalgic longing, a feeling of almost physical emptiness. Sometimes a memory of lost happiness is in the foreground of the depression, for instance, when it appears in the guise of an unhappy love experience. In other cases rage is the most important factor. A detailed investigation of these psychic mechanisms and of the causative factors can contribute more to the diagnosis than setting up twenty odd forms of depression. There is nevertheless no objection to distinguishing certain specific types of depression. One must bear in mind that many transitional forms occur and that a number of factors determine the manifestations of depression.

We can make our review of the depressions more poignant by comparing their manifestations with reactions of normal people. How does a healthy person react to an injury? There are different possibilities. As Freud pointed out, loss of a beloved person is followed by the work of mourning. To mourn is to detach oneself in gratitude for what the lost person has given us so that we may continue to pursue our way in life. However, when we are disappointed or angered by the person we have lost, other reactions take place. A different kind of psychic effort has to be undertaken. It is no less painful than loss of a beloved object. When disappointed, the normal person develops resentment and anger. He recognizes the other person's failings. When the situation permits it he expresses the anger, and simultaneously appeals to the other to alter his behavior. If the appeal is in vain he is capable of separating from the offending person. A mature adult will not seek revenge but will break off the relationship. Such action is impossible for someone whose ties to the object are infantile. To be adult implies to have power over one's aggression, to possess a healthy propensity for self-preservation, to be self-reliant, and not dependent on love of others for the bolstering of one's self-esteem. Hostile feelings are the fire which consumes the relationship to others; the adult person rises phoenixlike out of the ashes of his broken relationships.

As his life continues on its course he can observe tolerantly that the offender could not help being what he is. But one can achieve that detachment only when the disappointing relationship has been truly resolved. A pretense of having reached this attitude indicates inhibited aggression rather than psychic health. In depression the adult position gets lost through malignant regression to the patterns of symbiotic dependence.

What precipitates regression? It is frequently the injurious event itself, although neurotic conflict situations of various origin can also act as precipitating factors. Detailed examination of the life pattern of depressed patients indicates that even before the onset of their depression many of them had made use of unusual patterns of adaptation. They had never reached true inner independence; their oedipal problems had already precipitated regressive manifestations. Their self-esteem is extraordinarily dependent on praise, approval and affection. They tend to develop symbiotic patterns in their love relationships; to be loved for them means to be fed with love. Depression sets in when the mother-child relationship can no longer be continued, and when the emotional protection and approbation of such a relationship cease to surround them. The depression brings to light what has always been in existence although evident only to the careful observer. A much too dependent attitude was present through life, and the depression is the consequence of feeling abandoned and the inability to cope with this feeling. The vulnerability of depressive people is often accompanied by hidden fantasies of grandeur. As Lampl-de Groot (1927) has pointed out, these fantasies are meant to compensate for injuries. In reality they render the person even more vulnerable and susceptible to injury. Such persons expect to be treated by their environment in accordance with their fantasied image of themselves. They are given to characteristic attempts to solve conflict situations by submission and subservience. They lack capacity for productive rivalry and they avoid all struggles. Their self-confidence is shaky; it does not rest on an awareness of their own performance, but on approbation of others. Work is used as a means to earn praise and provides little or no healthy functional pleasure. The depressive person feels well when he is successful in finding security in the relationship with his spouse, and in gaining praise from his superiors. I have referred to this form of adaptation as "passive adaptation." These people are passive in the sense of being overly dependent and also in the sense of relying on gratification of drives with a passive aim. In their sexual life they are receivers rather than givers. Their inclination to avoid competition and rivalry with persons of the same sex, and their willingness to submit to them implies passive homosexual tendencies. This form of passivity easily turns into masochism. Depression appears when passive adaptation fails. It is possible to recognize the passive adaptation in the patient's history. It does, of course, also occur in neuroses free of depression.

Objections to the use of the term "passive adaptation" have been raised. It has been said that passivity implies the inability to be active. This, however, is not true. The people discussed above are at times capable of great efforts and considerable achievement. Their aim is nevertheless the passive gratification of being praised, appreciated and admired. The pattern of activity for the sake of a passive goal is well known. Freud has pointed out that women can be very active in their pursuit of gratification of drives with passive aims. "Passive" implies many things: to be dependent like an infant; to avoid competition and fight by submission; to strive for sublimated or direct sexual gratifications with a passive aim. I have chosen the term passive adaptation because it is clearly evident that an adult can have an instinctual organization identical with than of an infant. The physical and mental development may remain unaffected by the regression.

It should be stressed that the fateful element is not passive adaptation (which may at times be quite successful) but the reaction of the person to its failure. Loss of a mothering figure deprives the patient of needed support and attention, the depression develops as a reaction to that loss. The complementary etiological series of the causative factors in neurotic development demonstrated by Freud applies also in depressions. Often these people seem to be afflicted with a specific emotional vulnerability, and loss of security and care is pathogenic even for them.

What causes passive adaptation and how does it develop? In some cases the person holds onto and never progresses beyond early infantile preoedipal passivity—an arrest in development has occurred. In others, regression to the symbiotic pattern has occurred in order to avoid oedipal problems.

Since the Oedipus complex has not been optimally resolved, are the sexual functions not also impaired? As we have learned in the study of obsessive neurotic phenomena, disturbances in the oedipal period need not necessarily result in frigidity or impotence. In depression the situation is similar. The pathology involves self-esteem and self-assertion more than genital sexuality, though some involvement of sexuality is always present owing to dominance of drives with passive aim. The man does not derive sufficient gratification from an actively wooing position and the woman fails to derive satisfaction from an actively caring and protecting attitude. Sexual and narcissistic gratifications are not sufficiently separated. Self-esteem is too dependent on love and appreciation supplied by others.

It must further be pointed out that depression and depressive reactions occur simultaneously with many other neurotic symptoms. The anxiety of the depressed is as a rule a fear of being abandoned. Castration anxiety is also frequently present. Paranoid and hypochondriacal elaboration of guilt feelings and masochistic elaboration of passive sexuality are not uncommon. Sometimes depersonalization and derealization are used to ward off the depression and at times a deep depression is concealed by the sensation of not being able to feel anything at all. It must be emphatically pointed out that neurotic depressions with clearly understandable motivations are no less serious illnesses than endogenous depressions. There is often serious danger of suicide.

In investigating the depressions it must be kept in mind that the depressed mood is determined by mental as well as somatic factors. Unconscious emotional conflicts supply the roots for some depressions; in others the decline in the person's mood is caused by organic processes. From the examination of the neurasthenic syndrome we have learned that mood alterations are influenced by biological factors. We observed the coexistence of listlessness and hypersensitivity towards environmental and emotional stimuli. There is also a listlessness in connection with diminished sensitivity and a low level of emotionality. The sensation of no longer feeling anything may point to a mood alteration of vegetative origin. I should like to emphasize that such biological mood swings are by no means identical with a full-blown endogenous melancholia. The distinction is essential, and yet it is much too rarely taken into consideration. Van Praag (1962) published a paper which contains a number of accurate phenomenological distinctions. He lists the following symptoms of the biological depressive syndrome:

(1) Depressed mood, absence of zest, shrinking expectations in life, no adequate motives for the ill humor, which appears detached from its original motivation. The vague

incomprehensible feelings of discontent in the beginning are experienced as *lebensnah,* as close to life.

(2) Inhibition of thought and action, which is objectively observable or is experienced subjectively only.

(3) A diminished capacity to absorb affectively charged stimuli: "I can no longer enjoy anything." In the beginning of the illness it is primarily the stimuli which until then had been positvely charged that are so affected. The diminished sensitivity results in a loss of interest in relationships and activities which the patient had favored in the past.

(4) Disturbances of the time sense. The passage of time is experienced as slower than before the onset of the illness.

(5) Physical complaints such as loss of appetite, sleep disturbances, and fatigue in the absence of activity that could have caused it.

(6) These symptoms are most intense in the morning hours and diminish in intensity in the course of the day.

I am not convinced that diminished expectations in life and inhibition belong to the syndrome, they are symptoms of depression. In my opinion the following manifestations are part of the vegetative mood alteration syndrome: lassitude, fatigue, dullness, diminished sensitivity and emotionality, physical complaints like sleep disturbances, constipation, lack of appetite and changes of mood all in the course of the day.

Van Praag (1962) uses the term inhibition too broadly. Patients with neurotic depressions also feel inhibited and they too are subject to an attitude of hopelessness. Much more detailed research is necessary to decide whether such symptoms are expressions of a variation in biological vitality or neurotic manifestations. People who have recovered from a period of diminished vitality remark on their regained zest for life, and report that the intensity of experience has regained its former level. Depression is not always present in the loss-of-vitality syndrome.

Let us recapitulate the psychic mechanisms leading to

depressive reactions: (1) frustration of the passive need for love; (2) inhibition of aggression; (3) frustration of the fantasies of grandeur.

In depressive people conscious perception and expression of aggressive impulses are blocked. Helpless rage, obstinate rebellion, fantasies of grandeur and of omnipotence, rivalry and jealousy are repressed. As a rule biological variations in vitality result in a depression when neurotic problems become attached to them, and a mutually aggravating interchange ensues. It is this reciprocal vicious circle effect which causes the profound depressive reactions. The reverse, i.e., the precipitation of variations in vitality by a neurotic conflict occurs as well. In short, the somatic mental areas of the human organism are in constant interaction.

The separation of the syndrome of variations in vitality[1] from depression accompanied by disturbances of vitality finds confirmation in psychoanalytic experience. After the neurotic problems of patients suffering from cyclical depressions are resolved, the depression disappears, but variations in vitality persist. The lassitude and apathy no longer turn into a loathing of the future.

These considerations are of interest not only for the phenomenologist, but also for the practitioner. The struggle against depression has to be carried out on two fronts. When a neurotic depression has become paired with lowered vitality this component must also be treated.

For practical purposes the following division seems advisable: variations in vitality, depression with a component of such variations, neurotic depression resulting in disturbances of vitality. The treatment procedure should take the specific symptomatology into consideration. In deciding on the treatment method, one should consider variations in vitality, anxi-

---

[1] The term vitality as used here refers to the somatic aspect of life processes.

ety, agitation, hypochondriasis, paranoid manifestations, and catatonic traits. These subjects are comprehensively discussed in appropriate chapters of the related psychiatric literature. The description of symptoms in connection with an evaluation of different etiological factors is the most meaningful diagnostic approach. It provides the best insight into the disease processes and also indicates guidelines for therapy.

Finally, some observations about the prevention of depressions.

A society which demands that its members be not only valiant but warlike, cannot but subject many of them to the kind of traumatic situations which result in depressions. Goethe's sentiment that "man is either the hammer or the anvil" is still valid. The most gifted and therefore the most sensitive members of the society often are forced into the role of the anvil.

Problems in the early infantile situation, like those caused by an ambivalent attitude of a mother towards her child, initiate difficulties in the resolution of later problems. These in turn create an inclination to regression. A type of child rearing which prevents the child from integrating his instinctual impulses will encourage the tendency towards regression and the formation of neuroses. Too much frustration in early childhood creates an attitude of basic mistrust; overindulgence in later stages deprives the child of an opportunity to develop into a self-confident, strong adult. The attempt of many mothers to bring up their children as little saints often results in the child's developing an inclination to depressive reactions. The "good" child, so often held out as an example, is frequently a neurotic child. Too-ready compliance and submission to parental prohibitions and commands may be signs of the child's resorting to passive adaptation. These etiological factors direct our efforts at prevention of depressive illness. Mothers who love life in spite of its unavoidable disappointments and its suffering, possess the inner freedom to accept their child with a minimum of ambivalence. They are not hostile to the instinctual needs of their children and do not object to their children's sex. Such mothers can bring up children free from depression.

Situational factors may lead to a decompensation of passive adaptation and hence to mood anomalies. Some authors call such a depression reactive, others speak of a reactive depression when the depressive phase of a manic-depressive psychosis represents a response to a psychic trauma in a broad sense. Terminology is a matter of usage. Intensification of guilt feelings, loss of love, the breaking up of an ambivalent relationship and similar events can precipitate a depression. Variations in biological vitality must not be overlooked. However, I have seen depressions which had been diagnosed as endogenous, and were in reality reactions to an unbearable increase in unconscious guilt feelings. Without wishing to deny the significance of biologically caused variations in mood, I must emphasize that it is the neurotic problems, such as frustration of passive needs and poorly integrated aggression, which create a depression out of a biologically determined mood. When the biological decline levels off a precarious equilibrium is sometimes reestablished spontaneously. The course is difficult to predict because of the intimate interaction between endogenous and environmental factors.

There also occur chronically depressed character neuroses, the depression being their nuclear symptom. This aspect of character armor is as a rule extremely rigid. The different neurotic characters respond differently to injurious influences. Decompensation of the lonely sensitive character and an increased feeling of helplessness and fatigue in the neurasthenic character, are often accompanied by depression. All neurotics inclined to depressive reactions are particularly dependent on appreciation by and the good will of the environment.

ADDICTION

Narcissistic and libidinal gratifications characteristically coincide in addiction. The drug gratifies libidinal needs and enhances the self-esteem, albeit in a regressive manner. It is therefore natural to connect addiction with the phases of early infantile development. The oral character, the depressive and the addict use their relations with the environment for libidinal and narcissistic purposes simultaneously. We termed this feature a "malignant regression." Fenichel referred to people prone to depressive patterns as "love-addicts." Receiving of love and affection gratifies their libidinal needs and enhances their self-esteem; it provides them with the feeling that they are worthwhile persons. The addict is gratified by the introduction of a substance into his body which is ultimately detrimental to body and mind. Though the depressed patient is too dependent on receiving love, not all forms of this ambivalent love are detrimental to mental health. The person who has succeeded in the passive adaptation can establish relations with his environment which provide him with gratifications, he does not have to seek solace and support in the addictive substance. His instinctual gratifications remain on the genital level, though the genitality is predominantly passive. The behavior of the addict is determined by a much more extensive regression, and often normal sexual gratification has no significance for the addict at all. The ego of the depressed is, and the ego of the addict is not capable of avoiding the recourse to drugs. In regard to the connections between depression and addiction it is noteworthy that an addiction often serves to ward off feelings of depression, and it is almost always used to support the struggle against feelings of loneliness and despondency. Recourse to the drug is appealing because it is capable of temporarily enhancing self-esteem, counteracting feelings of despondency, and preventing anxiety, along with providing regressive libidinal gratifications. At times addiction is called upon to combat conscious feelings of dejection and sometimes the depression is warded off, i.e., the conscious awareness of depression is prevented with the help of the addiction. Addicts, like all people employing a passive adaptation and engaging in fantasies of grandeur, are very sensitive to injuries. Their excessively demanding ego ideals inevitably cause disappointments that lead to their seeking solace in alcohol and other addictive substances. As a rule their superegos are quite severe and induce the egos to an excessive defense against aggressive and infantile sexual tendencies. Addictive drugs mitigate the exacting demands of the superego. This is illustrated by the saying that the superego is "soluble" in alcohol. The superego is also "soluble" in amphetamines and opiates.

Love addiction and drug addiction differ significantly in their secondary effects. Except for the incidence of venereal infection sexual gratification is generally harmless, and certainly does not result in damage to ego functions. The somatic effect of drug addiction does, however, lead to an impairment of the functions of the ego. Frustration tolerance and capacity to postpone instinctual gratification are, to begin with, poorly developed in addicts. They are further weakened, and somatic factors are added to the neurotic vicious circle. The unavoidable hangover is unbearable, the old problems banned during the intoxication reappear in force, and with them emerge guilt feelings and a further diminution of self-esteem. The patient then seeks comfort in more alcohol, morphine or other drugs. Addicts are always in danger of passing from the category of the neuroses into the realm of organic disorders. Chronic alcoholism and delirium tremens are outside the scope of our discussion.

Much has been written about alcoholism. We are concerned with the abuse, not the use, of alcohol. This distinction has to be emphasized particularly by those who profess a belief in the Aristotelian "meson" which represents the result of an optimal integration. It is another matter that often "use" is referred to when "abuse" would be the correct term.

Manifestations of alcohol addiction are in many respects typical for oral regression. Alcohol provides oral libidinal gratification in the narrow and the broader sense of the term. The infant enjoys satiation and also the warmth supplied by the mother. The drinking of alcohol gives oral gratification and also a sensation of warmth through the dilatation of the peripheral vessels. References to alcohol as poisoned mother's milk evoke laughter, but the meaning is clearly understood. Alcohol grants the same satisfaction which the mother's milk gave to the nurseling, but ultimately the effect is harmful. Addiction is a form of masochistic self-destruction.

Addiction also often serves the purpose of permitting perverse fantasies to emerge into consciousness. Under the influence of alcohol people more readily accept their homosexual tendencies. It is interesting to note how often drinking together is a preliminary to the establishment of homosexual relations. The intoxicated friend is put to bed and, the resistance of the superego having been weakened by the alcohol, sleeping together follows. Western man pays dearly for his platonic attitude. Brought up to ward off drives, when he is inclined to satisfy an instinctual wish, even one sublimated in friendship or companionship, he must numb his superego with the help of some toxic drug. In Western Europe the rituals practiced in the name of friendship pave the way for the abuse of alcohol. Many students became uncertain and confused by acquiring new behavior patterns which conflict with their old ego ideal and superego standards. Insecurity engendered by a neurotic conflict frequently provides motivation for the abuse of alcohol. Insecure people often become authoritarian when intoxicated, bullying their children and causing neurotic behavior to develop.

The situational or social drinker need not be an alcoholic.

The need to be accepted into the group and not remain an outsider is in these cases responsible for occasional excesses. A true alcoholic is a person who is driven to the addiction by his unconscious conflicts, not by social motivations. The path to alcoholism may be made easier by the group which encourages drinking in certain situations. Drinking companions assist the drinker on the way to self-destruction, not to maturity. Conflict situations leading to alcholism are: Frustrated expectations, fantasies of grandeur, lack of the capacity for constructive rivalry, homosexual problems, inhibitions and work disturbances.

One of my patients began to drink heavily after his mother forbade him to continue a relationship with a pretty salesgirl. Homosexual inclinations were intensely warded off. During analytic treatment he succeeded in working through his negative Oedipus complex, his addiction disappeared, and he became able to take a social drink without losing control of himself. People free of conflicts motivating the addiction need not be phobic about alcohol.

Opiates take one into a dream world in which fantasy miraculously becomes reality. Infantile sexual wishes and their derivatives come to the fore. One must never disregard the social factors in addiction. People who live in a world of constant hunger, of poverty without prospect of improvement, understandably may wish to provide themselves with a happy dream.

Addictive stimulants differ in their effects from those of alcohol and morphine in the following ways: the stimulants do not immediately damage ego functions; they do not cause drowsiness and coma, like alcohol; they are taken to combat fatigue and sleepiness. The user feels that they alert his thinking and clear his mind. A euphoric mood makes its appearance and stays within tolerable limits if the dosage is kept within reason. However, many who take the common amphetamine tablets or a related drug feel restless and driven in spite of the improved mood. Undoubtedly people inclined to despondent reactions can experience a mood lift on taking a stimulant drug. The ego experiences the self with increased clarity. However, the actual performance frequently indicates that there is a dulling of awareness and of insight. Self-critical faculties are impaired, mistakes and incorrect conclusions are common. One can observe this readily during examinations of students who have taken stimulants. People who take stimulating drugs in order to remain alert on a long automobile trip actually drive less efficiently and are prone to accidents. The greatest fault of stimulants is that their effect is short-lived, and that repeated and larger doses are required. The frequent result is excessive fatigue with traits of the hypersensitive syndrome. Then follows a drop in mood which is usually deeper than the original reaction. A further unpleasant side effect is insomnia. Despondent people cannot bear sleeplessness and take sedatives which make them drowsy the next day. They take stimulants to combat the drowsiness. The physiological sleep rhythm is disturbed and replaced by a stimulant-hypnotic rhythm, very much to the detriment of the organism. Overdosage with stimulants results in unpleasant and dangerous physical and mental symptoms. Psychotic manifestations with hallucinations and paranoid imagery is not uncommon. It is wise to exercise great caution in prescribing stimulants. Barbiturate addiction, like addiction to opiates, aims to substitute fantasy for reality.

There are a number of harmless addictions, which show compulsive traits and to which Fenichel rightly called attention. Many people, for example, are addicted to travel, although the journey does not offer these "horizon hunters" relaxation but only escape from an inner emptiness. The collector may be another harmless addict, as well as the success-seeker. Many frustrated people seek solace in eating sweets in large quantities; the "obesity of grief" is a common phenomenon. Some people are helped during a decline in mood by reading. It is as though the mother were again reading to them and helping them to regain a feeling of security. Some hobbies have an addictive character. Much could be said about the psychology of hobbies. Undoubtedly there are connections between certain hobbies and solutions of instinctual problems. There is hardly anything that one can not become addicted to. Whether the respective activity assumes pathologic significance or represents a healthy attempt to self-cure depends on its function in the adaptation. Are these activities distracting attention from the problem, or do they contribute to its solution? The intensity and the quality of the respective activity determines whether it should be considered a normal or pathological phenomenon.

It is almost impossible to describe the course of an addiction. In order to make a prognostic evaluation one has to know a great deal more about the personality than the mere fact that addiction is present. If the addiction dominates the person's life, the condition is serious and requires intervention. As has been pointed out the use of drugs eventually damages those functions of the ego which must be mobilized to overcome the addiction. The patient has to learn to tolerate frustrations and to renounce some gratifications.

During difficult periods of life some people take refuge in the use of alcohol or drugs, and they overcome the habit when their circumstances have improved and the tensions subsided. Epilepsy can be accompanied by periodic episodes of abuse of alcohol, while depressions may be concurrent with periods of drug addiction. Evaluation of these manifestations also requires knowledge of the person's life history, personality, capacity for sublimation and his current circumstances. Early treatment of conditions of psychic tension is of great significance for the prevention of addictions.

9

TRAUMATIC NEUROSIS

EVERY neurosis is in a sense traumatic since it represents a disturbance in adaptation resulting from a trauma. The term traumatic neurosis was originally applied to neurotic reaction caused by events like overwhelming fright, sudden tragic misfortune, "shell shock," witnessing of fatal accidents and narrow escape from great danger. More recently the concept has been expanded to include reactions to physical injuries, reactions to excessive mental stress, and the pension neurosis.

In cases of neurotic reactions occurring after an accident careful examination of possible somatic etiological factors is mandatory. The neurosis can appear either directly in conjunction with the trauma, shortly after the patient emerges from the unconscious state, or after a long time interval. Fenichel (1931) lists the following manifestations: disturbances of ego functions, sleep disturbances, attacks of great anxiety, episodes of rage, repetitive reliving of the traumatic situation, and other neurotic symptoms.

When one imagines what it means to witness a comrade torn to pieces by an explosion, or to see one's friend swept into the abyss by an avalanche, it appears more appropriate to inquire how one can ever overcome such an experience than to search for the factors causing a traumatic neurosis.

The disturbance of ego function manifests itself in loss of interest in the environment. This is perhaps due to a change in energy distribution; all available energy is required for mastery of the traumatic experience. When an accident results in cerebral dysfunction and in simultaneous psychic trauma, it is often very difficult to determine the relative contributions of the two factors to the ego disturbance. It is understandable that a person who has suffered serious bodily injury or the loss of a beloved person tends to repress all content related to the painful experience.

Manifestations of pseudo mental deficiency can appear as symptoms of a traumatic neurosis. Sleep disturbances are caused by the inability to relax. The fear of remembering or of dreaming about the catastrophic event prevents relaxation and sleep.

The reliving of the traumatic event has been the object of much speculation, and has led to far-reaching theoretical conclusions. The tendency to re-experience the anxiety-provoking events seems to contradict the Aristotelian idea that man always strives to obtain happiness. It also contradicts Freud's original libido theory. However, the reliving of the anxiety-provoking situation can serve to master the anxiety and trauma. Consider the psychology of an exciting motion picture thriller. The viewer experiences true anxiety, with appropriate somatic symptoms. His heart pounds, he breaks out in sweat, but these unpleasant sensations do not prevent him from seeing the next thriller. On the contrary, these experiences act as a motive to see many more Hitchcock pictures or similar productions. The explanation is as follows: the viewer experiences the fact that he can bear the anxiety and its quick disappearance with pleasure. It is gratifying and encouraging. The biological rationale for seeking out an anxiety-producing situation is the mastery of the anxiety. This promotes a feeling of well-being, and even some pleasure. The little child raised high by the father's strong arms shouts with joy, he is no longer afraid of the height. By our analogy we do not intend to make little of the intense suffering of the patient with a traumatic neurosis. It serves merely to point out the element of mastering the anxiety. The attempt to master a situation is not the only reason for the repetition compulsion. Someone with intense feelings of guilt and a corresponding need for punishment will perceive the trauma as a just punishment and a necessary penance for his misdeeds. The punitive superego compels the ego to relive the unhappy experience again and again.

One often sees depressive manifestations in the context of a traumatic neurosis. Fenichel (1931) has pointed out that the soldier is forced into a dependent situation. He expects protection from his superior officers. When he discovers in the course of battle that these figures are quite unable to protect him, an overwhelming feeling of abandonment overpowers him, and a clincial condition reminiscent of the anaclitic depression develops. Along with the fear of loneliness and abandonment, castration anxiety is activated; many traumatic neuroses consequently show similarities with nontraumatic neurotic illness. Bastiaans (1957) has pointed out that many traumatic neuroses begin with neurasthenic symptoms, and these manifestations then dominate the course of the neurosis. The course depends on the kind of treatment the patient receives. He must be helped to recognize the physical causes of his complaints. This gives him some feeling of certainty about his condition. The patient is entitled to this information, although harsh attitudes of physicians and medical authorities have forced patients into an attitude of resistance because this information was withheld. Because it is an insult to the patient to be accused of pretending to be ill, he is forced to emphasize his complaints in order to convince the doctor, which in turn serves to confirm in the doctor's view that the patient is malingering. The symptoms may be psychogenic in nature; they are, nonetheless, manifestations of disease. Nobody is mentally disturbed for the pleasure of it, and nobody values a pension higher than the ability to be productive.

The therapy of traumatic neurosis is outside the scope of this book, but I should like, nevertheless, to point out that many difficulties arise out of a mistaken attitude of the therapist in early stages of the illness. Bastiaans has put together the symptoms occurring in the traumatic neuroses in the following way: The first stage is that of shock, in which loss of consciousness is the dominant symptom. The next stage, shock-counter-shock-alarm, shows much similarity with the neurasthenic syndrome. There follows a stage of defense reactions, which are characterized by a "flight or fight" attitude or by a simultaneous presence of both reactions. The type of reaction depends on the premorbid personality structure. In the "fighting" character, open hostility, cynicism and destructive criticism prevail, while the "flight" characters are indifferent, discouraged and apathetic. These symptoms are reminiscent of the neurasthenic triad of listlessness, hopelessness, and helplessness.

PENSION NEUROSIS

Traumatic neurosis and the pension neurosis are understandably described in conjunction, since both develop in connection with a traumatic event. The patient with a pension neurosis is unable to overcome the real or unreal results of a physical injury, he wants to be compensated for it. Often the neurosis follows a concussion syndrome; dizziness, fatigue, sleep disturbances and headache in the wake of a concussion can provide a factor of "somatic compliance," and become neurotically fixated. Hysterical neurasthenic syndromes and paranoid elaborations occur in persons afflicted with pension neurosis. Passive forms of adaptation are common. Their history indicates a preference toward infantile solutions of life problems and a dependent and demanding attitude. A typical complaint: "I have always done my best, and now I am dropped because I can't perform as well any more, and the fact that the accident happened at work counts for nothing."

The masochistic attitude gratifies the need for punishment, as well as the neurotically elaborated passive homosexual needs. The partial loss of the capacity to work represents for some people an injury to their self-esteem. The patient demands that society compensate him for this injury. Fortunately the time is past when the doctor blamed the patient for malingering when an attempt at diagnosis failed to reveal an organic basis for the patient's complaints. The transition between conscious and unconscious is sometimes gradual, and some conversion symptoms express what is not entirely conscious. I cannot caution too much against simplification of psychic phenomena which takes easy recourse to the diagnosis of malingering. To declare someone a malingerer on the basis of his apparent dislike of work indicates a regrettable lack of insight and/or compassion. In these cases a heavy responsibility to prevent injustice and unnecessary suffering rests on the examining physician. The psychic mechanisms in the pension neurosis are the same as in other neurotic conditions. One must pay particular attention to the possibility of organic disease, and be guided by the reconstruction of the genesis and the dynamics of the case.

10

<hr>

THE PERVERSIONS

WE CAN describe perversions as pathological deviations of sexual behavior in which certain sexual desires—for example, exhibitionism, voyeurism, sadism, masochism, homosexuality, and fetishism—are acted out. We must always remember that our primary concern is with people, with suffering patients, and only secondarily are we interested in dynamic connections and mechanisms.

The study of people with perversions discloses that we can distinguish two main groups among them, with transitional groupings between the two groups. One group is related to the neuroses, the other to the psychopathies. As we have described previously the neurotic has a more serviceable super-ego and a healthier ego ideal than the psychopath. The ego functions of the psychopathic personality are deficient. These distinctions may be useful in our examination of the perversions.

We know patients who suffer intensely because they have perverse fantasies, and almost never act them out in reality. If they behave in accordance with their fantasies they feel extremely guilty whether their action is discovered or not. We know homosexuals who do not satisfy their needs because they suffer from feelings of guilt and the fear of injuring the other person. The shy and self-conscious exhibitionist tries desperately to resist the pressure of his desire, until he can no longer control his tension, and exhibits his penis to a girl passing by. There are, however, also different types of homosexual patients, who aggressively seek out objects for their gratification and have little or no concern for the serious damage they may inflict on some preadolescent boy.

The psychiatrist engaged in the examination of perverse people under sentence by a court is familiar with some who do not suffer from their perversion, but fear the punishment of the law. What appears to be a feeling of guilt is in reality social anxiety. The suffering of these people is not the result of their perversion, but of its discovery by the authorities. The perversions of the neurotic group are more amenable to treatment than those of the psychopathic group. One seldom sees people of the psychopathic group in treatment. They seek it only when under court order, or when they fear the police.

The common denominator of all perversions, precisely described by Freud (1905), are the deviations in the aim and object of the sexual drive. I quote once again from the *Three Essays on Sexuality:* "let us call the person from whom sexual attraction proceeds the *sexual object,* and the act towards which the instinct tends the *sexual aim*" (pp. 135–136). In pedophilia, children replace the adult sexual object; in sodomy, animals; in necrophilia, a dead person. In these perversions, the sexual aim is unchanged; orgasm. Examples of deviations in regard to the sexual aim include exhibitionism, voyeurism, sadism, and masochism. Freud's formulations in this respect have retained their validity. In my opinion it is descriptively and phenomenologically incorrect to place homosexuality on the same level with sodomy or necrophilia. The psychological significance of a sexual relationship with a friend differs markedly from that with an animal or a corpse. Necrophilia and sodomy can hardly be ego-syntonic phenomena, but a homosexual relationship with a friend can be ego-syntonic. Although homosexuality is frowned upon by Western standards, passive feminine wishes are universal. Their elaboration may, of course, differ from case to case. We see the relationship between neurosis and perversion differently from Freud. He formulated the description which created much puzzlement: "Neurosis is the negative of perversion." We can express it thus: What is acted out in a perversion is repressed in neurosis. An example: Neurotic self-consciousness, stammering and blushing of a man in the presence of a woman may be based on the warded-off wish to impress her with his penis. In perversion this wish is acted out: The man exposes his penis. What is expressed with this action? Freud's reply to this question was: A component drive, i.e., an immature component of the sexual drive. Component drives can acquire dominant significance in sexual life. In such a case the aim of the sexual drive is not orgasm but the wish to see, to be looked at, to touch and be touched, to inflict or suffer pain.

Current literature emphasizes the defense function of the perversion. The perverse actions are more than expressions of component drives, they serve to ward off other instinctual impulses. The principle of stratification of the defensive processes is important for the comprehension of all psychic disturbances, and particularly for the treatment of perversion. Freud at first believed that perversions were not treatable. Wilhelm Reich (1933), in particular, demonstrated the stratified structure of the defense processes. That knowledge can be applied successfully to the therapy of perversions. The perverse patient gratifies an instinctual impulse and thereby wards off anxiety. The nature of the warded-off anxiety becomes evident when we combine genetic and dynamic approaches.

Before continuing with this subject, I should like to call attention to a further feature of perverse sexuality, that is, its mode of experience (Kronfeld, 1930). This feature has received more attention from clinical psychiatrists than from analysts. My teacher, a psychiatrist of rich experience, has repeatedly pointed out that the position of perverse sexuality within the total personality is different from that of normal sexuality. Perverse drives are more demanding; the mode of experience is addictive. Since perverse actions are repeated with a compulsive intensity one may think of a compulsive neurosis; yet, persons with perversions do not experience them as compulsions, though the neurotic perversions may be perceived as ego alien. Fenichel's (1945) formulation is quite accurate: "The compulsive neurotic feels compelled to do things which he dislikes doing, i.e., he must pit his will-power against his wishes; the pervert feels compelled to like something against his will." Sometimes even genital sexuality is experienced in a manner which reminds the observer of an addiction; Le Coultre (1956) wrote of cases of genital perversion.

The defensive function of perverse sexuality gives it its compelling character. The perverse experience wards off other strivings and anxieties; a function which the perversion is called upon constantly to perform so that the other tendencies may remain safely repressed. The same applies to those forms of sexual life which, though they retain normal aim and object, appear to have an excessive intensity of drive. An example of this type is the "Don Juan" character which, in common with perversion, has the impulse-driven aspect of behavior.

Let me summarize our ideas about Freud's thesis that neurosis is the negative of perversion. The perverse impulse, like the hysterical, has a defensive component, which explains the addictive character of the perverse person's "mode of experience." For some time I thought that all perversions displayed this dynamic feature. This idea proved very fruitful as a working hypothesis. Lampl-de Groot (1927) believes that some perverse persons suffer from a primary disturbance of the drive organization.

It is possible that the sadist has to render his victim help-less in order to ward off anxiety, or that he has to destroy because he fears castration. But it is also possible that the organization of his drive contains an innate anomaly. Only further research, not our more or less pessimistic views about human nature, will decide the issue. Undoubtedly, the ego idea and the ego functions will have to be reconsidered in this context. The question will have to be answered: Why does one man suffer from his perversion, while another man inflicts suffering on others?

Can the perversions be understood dynamically and genetically? It is not puzzling that one man receives ultimate gratification from a stocking, another from shoes with high heels and still another insists on being whipped with a riding crop held in red-gloved hands by a woman wearing leather rid-ing breeches? What drives these people?

The answer of psychoanalysis to this question is in my opinion one of its most significant findings. Before psycho-analysis, attempts were made to explain these phenomena as follows: The adolescent boy had seen the stocking on the sex-ually exciting leg of a woman and the stocking became the source of his sexual excitement. The masochistic man had been once beaten by his nurse, and therefore seeks out this form of gratification. Such a biographical or historical explanation disregards unconscious motivations and is not satis-factory. One must consider the unconscious factors. In-vestigation of these factors reveals that the patient with a perversion cannot tolerate the difference between the sexes. The fetishist is excited by something which belongs to the woman because he unconsciously perceives this object as the woman's penis. Her leg, her hands, her shoes calm his fears. When we listen to the language of his unconscious we per-ceive the assurance that woman, too, has that precious organ, that she is not mutilated. Masochistic man blurs the sexual distinction in this way: The red gloves and the leather riding breeches point to masculine sexual attributes, i.e., the sexual partner is given a symbolic penis.

While the fetishist and the masochist attribute masculine features to woman, homosexual man turns away from her entirely. He feels no passion for woman, a being without a penis.

The statement that the pervert cannot tolerate an object without a penis is particularly clearly exemplified by the active homosexual woman who uses a penis prosthesis to gratify her homosexual partner.

There are three possibilities for the relationship of man to woman: (1) The woman is experienced and valued as a woman. (2) The woman is rejected, because no being without a penis can be loved. (3) A penis is attributed to a penisless object, the fact of the absence of the penis is disavowed.

In cases of manifest bisexuality and passive adaptation in males we see an alternating pattern of choice of sexual object. A homosexual partner changes places with a "phallic" woman who is fantasied as possessing a penis. The emphasis in all such relationships is on the idea: We are entirely alike, and can do the same things. There are no men and women, all creatures are identical. Insofar as there are differences between them, it is not that one has something which the other lacks. Therefore one finds a predilection for being able to do the same thing together among the participants in different forms of perverse sexuality. This mutual experience of pregenital forms of sexuality is found in many perversions which have no specific name, for instance, urinating or defecating together. Even when the genital organs are drawn into the sexual activity there is still a preference for activities that can be "done together." The insistence of mutual masturbation instead of intercourse can be based on an unconscious disavowal or rejection of the difference between the sexes.

We are now prepared to recognize that the ultimate motivation of the perverse person, the springboard of his peculiar behavior, is the castration complex. The need to deny castration is paramount in his makeup. This realization enables us to bring perversion in connection with other deviating sexual behavior patterns that are usually not counted among perversions, for example, the tendency to enter triangular situations and promiscuity.

Castration anxiety is expressed in the following examples of perversion:

Voyeurism. The voyeur identifies with the female partner of the couple he observes in the sexual act, in this manner he has a partner who possesses a penis. Simultaneously, he is aroused by a woman who at the time of intercourse "possesses" a penis, that of her partner. It is clear that the negative Oedipus complex, passive homosexuality, and the need to endow woman with a penis all have their roots in castration anxiety.

Exhibitionism. The corresponding unconscious motivation of the exhibitionist can be expressed as follows: I am not castrated, I can show you that I am not, and I implore you to let me see that you are not castrated either.

Transvestitism. When I dress in woman's clothing I prove that a woman's dress contains a penis.

Masochism. A woman beats me, but she has male attributes, she is a man. Freud stated that the content of this fantasy is the wish to be forced into sexual submission by a man.

Sadism, and some forms of necrophilia. The woman is not dangerous, she cannot mutilate me or castrate me, I mutilate her.

Pregenital preferences. The predilection for pregenital forms of sexuality and for activities in which both partners can "do the same" denies differences between the sexes by asserting that what man can do to or with woman, she can do to or with man.

The problems connected with the sex differences are met differently by men and women. The disavowal of the sex difference is rare in woman. Perversions are consequently uncommon in women, but when they occur, the disavowal of the sex difference plays an important role, if not the most important role in their genesis. For example: A woman experiences intensive sexual arousal on imagining that her friend urinates while his penis is in her vagina. She tries to persuade him to do what excites her so much in fantasy. It is clear that her behavior is determined by the fantasy "I have a penis." This patient intensely desired to engage with her friend in pregenital activities, to urinate and defecate in his presence.

We have to examine what role the impulses which express themselves in the perversion play in normal life. It is a mark of Freud's genius that in his *Three Essays on Sexuality* he taught us to recognize the normal elements in manifestations of definitely abnormal behavior.

The component drives, exhibitionism, voyeurism, the pleasure in observing behavior connected with sexuality are being gratified in normal love-play preparatory to the sexual act. There exists a perfectly normal form of fetishism. Almost every man looks at a girl's legs, and many are stimulated by girls supplied with male attributes and attired in an imitation of male clothing, etc. Motion pictures and the advertising industry make liberal use of this fact. Long-legged women are considered particularly desirable.

Anality and orality may play a significant role in a sexual contact which nevertheless ends in a normal coitus; this pattern has the same meaning as the perversion. "We do the same things, we are not different from each other." However, if the orgasm is achieved normally, we do not term a pattern perverse.

Sadism and masochism are not disturbing if their intensity is not excessive. The criterion of a perversion is the inability to reach orgasm in the normal way and the preponderance of component drives, i.e., the sexual interest in nongenital areas of the body has failed to be integrated into the total sexual experience. Sometimes perverse needs persist in spite of a capacity for normal coitus. We must consider such a situation pathological. The prognosis of these conditions is favorable, the fixation to early stages being only partial.

We have explained the perversions based on unconscious disavowal of the difference of the sexes and on castration anxiety. In perversions which make use of surrogate objects, i.e., sodomy and pedophilia, misidentifications play the main role, rather than the mechanisms mentioned above.

Freud's statement that the Oedipus complex is the nucleus of the neuroses applies to the perversions which are structured like a neurosis. Castration anxiety causes abandonment of the appropriate normal object, and the intensity of the castration anxiety is conditioned by the Oedipus complex. Perversions are invariably connected with regressive processes related to and occasioned by unresolved oedipal problems. There are many reasons for the failure to resolve the Oedipus complex in a healthy manner. One of them which deserves mention is the large quantity of early childhood rage that has not been properly discharged, where intense ambivalence exists in association with the oedipal situation. The regression wards off not only the sexual, but also the aggressive impulses connected with the Oedipus complex.

With regard to the course of the perversions, it can be stated that the perverse needs increase in intensity when castration fears are warded off, or when aggressive impulses become more pressing. Some people find a way of adaptation and learn to live with their symptoms. At times the corresponding guilt feelings are more disturbing than the perverse symptom itself. It is difficult to decide how often homosexual relationships are gratifying and stable, since the psychiatrist sees only those cases in which the relationship has failed. For one person the perversion may be an alien element causing much distress, while another may find an adequate *modus vivendi.* Some people gratify perverse needs with prostitutes and retain a semblance of a normal sexual relationship within their marriage. This is at times the most practical solution achievable.

When the perversion causes a person to come in conflict with the law, his future life is significantly influenced. It must always be borne in mind that notwithstanding their general similarities, the perversions differ greatly in their significance and their effect on the life of the individual.

REFERENCES

Abraham, K. (1920), Manifestations of the Female Castration Complex. In: *Selected Papers.* London: Hogarth Press, 1948, pp. 338–369.

Bastiaans, J. (1957), Psychosomatische gevolgen van onderdrukking en verzet. Dissertation. Amsterdam.

Bergler, E. (1946), *Unhappy Marriage and Divorce: A Study of Neurotic Choice of Marriage Partners.* New York: International Universities Press.

Carp, E. A. D. E. (1947), *Die Neurosen* (3rd Ed.).

Chrzanowski, G. (1959), Neurasthenia and Hypochondriasis. In: *American Handbook of Psychiatry,* Vol. 1, ed. S. Arieti. New York: Basic Books, pp. 258–271.

Cleckley, H. (1955), *The Mask of Sanity.* St. Louis: C. V. Mosby.

————— (1959), Psychopathic States. In: *American Handbook of Psychiatry,* Vol. 1, ed. S. Arieti. New York: Basic Books, pp. 567–588.

Eissler, K. R., ed. (1949), Some Problems of Delinquency. In: *Searchlights on Delinquency.* New York: International Universities Press, pp. 3–25.

Erikson, E. H. (1950), *Childhood and Society.* New York: Norton.

Fenichel, O. (1931), Über Homosexualität. *Psychoanalytische Bewegung,* 3:511–526.

————— (1945), *The Psychoanalytic Theory of the Neuroses.* New York: Norton.

Freud, A. (1936), *The Ego and the Mechanisms of Defense.* New York: International Universities Press, rev. ed., 1966.

————— (1959), Paper read before the International Psychoanalytic Congress, Copenhagen.

Freud, S. (1894), Studies on Hysteria. *Standard Edition*, 2:1–310. London: Hogarth Press, 1955.

―――― (1905), Three Essays on Sexuality. *Standard Edition*, 7:125–230. London: Hogarth Press, 1953.

―――― (1908), Character and Anal Eroticism. *Standard Edition*, 9:167–177. London: Hogarth Press, 1959.

―――― (1909), Analysis of a Phobia in a Five-Year-Old Boy. *Standard Edition*, 10:5–147. London: Hogarth Press, 1955.

―――― (1912), On the Universal Tendency to Debasement in the Sphere of Love. *Standard Edition*, 11:177–190. London: Hogarth Press, 1957.

―――― (1916–1917), Introductory Lectures on Psycho-Analysis. *Standard Edition*, 16. London: Hogarth Press, 1963.

―――― (1918), From the History of an Infantile Neurosis. *Standard Edition*, 17:3–104. London: Hogarth Press, 1955.

―――― (1926), Inhibition, Symptom and Anxiety. *Standard Edition*, 20:87–173. London: Hogarth Press, 1959.

―――― (1931), Female Sexuality. *Standard Edition*, 21:223–243. London: Hogarth Press, 1961.

―――― (1933), New Introductory Lectures on Psycho-Analysis. *Standard Edition*, 22:31–182. London: Hogarth Press, 1964.

Frijung-Schreuder, E. C. M. (1964–1965), Honoré de Balzac. *Psyche*, 18:606–615.

Hartmann, H. (1939), *Ego Psychology and the Problem of Adaptation*. New York: International Universities Press, 1958.

Huehnerfeld, P. (1959), *In Sachen Heidegger*. Hamburg.

James, W. (1899), *Talks to Teachers on Psychology; and to Students on Some of Life's Ideals*. New York: Dover.

Johnson, A. M. (1949), Sanctions for Superego Lacunae of Adolescence. In: *Searchlights on Delinquency*, ed. K. R. Eissler. New York: International Universities Press, pp. 225–245.

Kraus, G. (1947), Verworven (postmorbide) psychopathieën. In: *Psychiatrische en neurologische bladen*, 50:417–436.

Kretschmer, E. (1927), *Der sensitive Beziehungswahn* (3rd ed.). Berlin: Springer, 1950.

Kroll, M. (1929), *Die Neuropathologischen Syndrome*. Berlin.

Kronfeld, A. (1930), *Die Perspectiven der Seelenheilkunde*. Leipzig: Thieme.

Kuiper, P. C. (1958), Onechtheid een neurotisch symptoom. *Ned. tijdschr. v. Geneesk*, 102.

———— (1961), Der negative Odipuskomplex beim Mann. In: *Jahrbuch der Psychoanalyse*, Vol II. Cologne: Westdeutcher Verlag, pp. 63–79.

Ladee, G. A. (1961), Hypochondrische Syndromen. Dissertation. Amsterdam.

Lampl-de-Groot, J. (1928), The Evolution of the Oedipus Complex in Women. *Internat. J. Psycho-Anal.*, 9:332–345.

Le Coultre, R. (1956), Elimination of Guilt as a Function of Perversions. In: *Perversions: Psychodynamics and Therapy*. New York: Random House, pp. 42–54.

Menninger, W. C. (1943), Characterologic and Symptomatic Expressions related to the Anal Phase of Development. *Psychoanal. Quart.*, 12:61–195.

Reich, W. (1933), *Character Analysis*. New York: Orgone Institute Press, 1945.

Van Dantzig, A. and Waage, J. (1962), Almacht en onmacht; het verband tussen psychasthenie en neurasthenie. *Huisarts en Wetenschap*.

Van der Waals, C. (1940), Narcistische Problematiek van het Narcisme. *Psychiatrische en Neurologische Bladen*, 44:537–628.

Van Praag, H. M. (1962), Een kritisch Onderzoek naar de betekenis van monoamine-oxydase-remming als therapeutisch principe bij de behandeling von depressies. Dissertation. Nijmegen.

Zutt, J. (1929), Die innere Haltung, eine psychologische Untersuchung usw. *Mtschr. Psychiatrie u. Neurologie*. 73:50, 243, 330.

INDEX

Abasia, hysterical, 99
Abdominal pains, 98, 99
Abraham, K., 72, 90, 93, 127, 128, 132, 136
Accidents, neurotic reactions to, 234–235
Acting out, in perversions, 88, 89
Adaptation
  and defense mechanisms, 26
  and disadaptation, 86
  ego ideal affecting, 40
  mechanisms in, 2–3, 67–68
  passive, 14, 26, 221–222, 228
  and pension neurosis, 237
  in sensitive characters, 172–173
  superego affecting, 40
Addiction, 89, 228–233
Adolescence, 65–66
  masturbation in; see Masturbation
  obsessive-compulsive neurosis in, 202
Affect
  compulsive, 184
  repression of, 23–24
Affective relationships in childhood, importance of, 8–9
Aggression against self, in depression, 211, 216, 218
Aggressive drive, 48
  and desire for punishment, 58
  inhibition of, 171–172
  in obsessive-compulsive neurosis, 190
  and projection, 18
Alcoholism, 229–231
Alloplastic reactions, 82–83, 133
Ambivalence, 50, 54–55
  and depression, 214
Anal phase of development, 47–51
  and frigidity, 103
  and obsessive-compulsive neurosis, 180, 186, 187, 189–192, 195

Anger
  in childhood, turned against oneself, 34–35, 36, 37
  and defense mechanisms, 34–35
  in depression, 216–218
  displacement of, 21–23
  at introjected object, 213–215, 218
Animals
  cruelty to, 190–191
  fear of, 108
Anxiety, 104–108
  in childhood, 19, 28–29
  and defense mechanisms, 19–20, 28–29, 106
  and depression, 223
  and hysteria, 104–108, 143, 162
  introjection of anxiety-provoking figures, 36–37
  mastery of, 235–236
  in neuroses, 106–107
  in oedipal phase, 55–56
  and organ-neurotic symptoms, 98
  pathological absence of, 105
  and perceptive function, 8
  and perversions, 241, 243
  and sadism, 243
Asceticism, in puberty, 64
Astasia, hysterical, 99
Asthenia, 201–202
Authority, conflict with, 78, 93, 154, 155
Autoplastic reactions, 82–83, 133

Backaches, 98
Barbiturate addiction, 232
Bastiaans, J., 199, 201, 236, 237
Bergler, E., 79, 103
Bisexuality
  manifest cases of, 244
  in obsessive-compulsive neurosis, 190
Blindness, hysterical, 99